# *Sources for prosexual drugs & nutrients*

Please copy this page mail it to us at: Smart Publications,™ POB 4667, Petaluma, CA 94955. We'll send you (free) our *Directory of Mail Order Pharmacies* (where you can buy many of the drugs & nutrients discussed in this book) plus our *Directory of Physicians* (which may help you find a knowledgeable and understanding doctor).

Name: _____

Company: _____

Address: _____

City/State/Zip: _____

Phone: _____

E-mail address (if any): _____

Online service (if any): _____

What magazines do you read: _____

_____

Age (optional): _____ Annual income (optional): _____

☐   I am a health professional. Please add me to your directory.

## Please rate the following items from 1 to 3.
(1 - high interest;  2 - moderate interest;  3 - no interest)

_____ A monthly newsletter covering smart drugs, prosexual drugs and life extension.

_____ Our personalized medical research service. (We do computer searches on your medical questions.)

_____ Order information for the other smart drugs books: *Smart Drugs & Nutrients* and *Smart Drugs II: The Next Generation.*

_____ A book on fat loss by the authors of this book.

_____ The pharmaceutical products discussed in this book.

_____ The nutritional supplement products discussed in this book.

_____ Order information for the products formulated by Durk Pearson & Sandy Shaw.

Nutritional formulations I'd like to see: _____

_____

# Books From Smart Publications™

## Smart Drugs & Nutrients
*How to Improve Your Memory And Increase Your Intelligence Using The Latest Discoveries in Neuroscience*
by Ward Dean, M.D., and John Morgenthaler
Smart Publications™ (formerly Health Freedom Publications) 1990
$12.95

## Smart Drugs II: The Next Generation
*New Drugs and Nutrients to Improve Your Memory and Increase Your Intelligence*
by Ward Dean, M.D., John Morgenthaler, and Steven Wm. Fowkes
Smart Publications™ (formerly Health Freedom Publications) 1993
$14.95

## Natural Hormone Replacement
*For Women Over 45*
by Jonathan V. Wright, M.D., and John Morgenthaler
$9.95

## GHB
*The Natural Mood Enhancer*
by Ward Dean, M.D., John Morgenthaler, and Steven Wm. Fowkes
$14.95

## STOP the FDA
*Save Your Health Freedom*
edited by John Morgenthaler and Steven Wm. Fowkes
Smart Publications™ (formerly Health Freedom Publications) 1992
$9.95

Smart Publications™
PO Box 4667 Petaluma, CA 94955

Phone: (707) 769-8308
On the Internet: http://www.smart-publications.com/smart

# What people said about
## *Smart Drugs & Nutrients* and
## *Smart Drugs II: The Next Generation*

"*...a fascinating and controversial subject...*"
**Barbara Walters, *ABC Nightline***

" *...a bible for the smart drug set.*"
**Los Angeles Times Magazine**

" *...an excellent introduction to the field of cognition-enhancing compounds... well-written and easily understood, even by people who do not have specific training in medicine.*"
**Giacomo Spignoli, M.D., Ph.D.**
**Pharmacology Research Director, L. Manetti-H. Roberts**

" *...a very important book. Very interesting and well documented...an absolutely essential and important subject.*"
**Timothy Leary, Ph.D.**

" *...a very interesting, well-researched book. Well done!*"
**Ross Pelton, R.Ph., Ph.D.**
**Author of *Mind Food And Smart Pills***

" *...a well-researched and referenced work...an antidote to the plethora of popular articles on intelligence enhancement that always seem to end by telling you that it's coming, but it'll be years before you can benefit from this technology...invaluable to people who want to take advantage of available intelligence enhancement technology now.*"
**Durk Pearson & Sandy Shaw**
**Authors of *Life Extension: A Practical Scientific Approach***

" *...it's enough to make Nancy Reagan just say yes.*"
*Playboy Magazine*

# Better Sex Through Chemistry

## A Guide to the New Prosexual Drugs

by John Morgenthaler & Dan Joy

Smart Publications™
PO Box 4667
Petaluma, CA 94955

Phone: (707) 769-8308
http://www.smart-publications.com/smart

*Better Sex Through Chemistry*
*A Guide to the New Prosexual Drugs*

**by John Morgenthaler & Dan Joy**

Published by:
Smart Publications™
PO Box 4667
Petaluma, CA 94955
Phone: (707) 769-8308
http://www.smart-publications.com/smart

Library of Congress Catalog Card Number: 94-74007
First Printing 1995
Printed in the United States of America
First Edition

Library of Congress Cataloging in Publication Data
Morgenthaler, John.
Better Sex Through Chemistry: A Guide to the New Prosexual Drugs
/ by John Morgenthaler and Dan Joy.
    Includes references and index.
    1. Sex (Biology)—Nutritional aspects.
    2. Sex.
    3. Neuropharmacology.
    4. Aging—prevention.
    5. Health.
QP251.W26    1994    613.9'5        93-22227
ISBN: 0-9627418-2-5:   $14.95 Softcover

10 9 8 7 6 5 4 3 2

# Acknowledgements

Special thanks go to the following individuals for their encourage-ment and thoughtful editorial feedback: Will Block; Jeremy Broner; Ward Dean, MD; Steven Fowkes; Lane Lenard; Samantha Miller; Dodson Miller Morgenthaler; Durk Pearson; Bill Powell; Sandy Shaw; Alexander T. Shulgin, PhD; and Lynn Ann Wilson.

We would also like to thank all those whose support made it possible for us to do this work including: Jeff Card; Hyla Cass, MD; Troy Dickerson; Wayne Morgenthaler; Sebastian Orfali; Beverly Potter; Gary Ross, MD; Jeremy Slate.

And, special thanks to: Shannon Boomer; Michael and Liza Brickey; Daniel Briggs; Brumbaer; Robin Christiensen; Fraser Clark & the staff of Megatripolis San Francisco; the Delay Family Robinson; Christopher Farabee; Marilyn Ferguson; Frode Holm; Jason Keehn; Timothy Leary; Mark Metz; Planet 6 Sound; Traci Ponciano; Scott Rossner; Robert Schulenberg; The "788" Club; Michael Siegel; Alex Strange; T.A.Z.; Tone Dog; Aaron Turner; Katlea Veridean; and Your Sisters' House.

**A note on the references:** We would like to thank all those scientists whose hard work this book is based on. In the text of this book we frequently cite scientific papers by giving the first author name and the date, for example "[Chin, 1992]." The full reference for those papers can be found in the back of this book where all the authors are listed (not just the first). We use this convention only for the sake of brevity and, most emphatically, wish to thank *all* the researchers whose work we cite.

To the best of our knowledge, the term "prosexual drugs" was first used by R.C. Rosen and A.K. Ashton in their excellent paper, "Prosexual Drugs: Empirical status of the 'new aphrodisiacs.'" We would like to thank Rosen and Ashton for providing us with this new term and thereby liberating us from the negative baggage attached to the word "aphrodisiac."

# Disclaimer

**Reader Please Note:** The material in this book has been collected and published for educational purposes only. It is not intended to provide medical advice. Please do not use the material in this book as a substitute for advice from your personal physician. If you wish to act on some information you find in this book, please consult with a knowledgeable physician. Do not try to be your own doctor.

There could be errors in this book. Although we have proofread this book many times, have had colleagues carefully check it, and we think it is quite accurate compared to other popular health books, there are probably still some errors. Please do not rely on this book as your sole reference source, especially with regard to dosages and contraindications.

It is not our intention to make any recommendations for the use of the substances discussed, nor do we wish to make any medical recommendations at all. We are not doctors. The information in this book is designed to provide you with hints about what to ask your doctor. Please consult a knowledgeable physician before putting any of the ideas in this book into practice.

# Table of Contents

# Introduction

This is a book of real, modern-day, pharmaceutical break-throughs for enhancing your sex life. These discoveries will benefit people in good sexual health as well as those with specific sexual dysfunctions. We believe that almost everyone can have better sex thorough the use of the new *prosexual* drugs and nutrients.

A prosexual drug or nutrient is any substance that can improve sex or sexual health. The compounds covered in this book can enhance sex drive, erection, frequency of orgasm, intensity of orgasm, stamina, vaginal lubrication, skin sensitivity, personal enjoyment of sex, and even intimacy and emotional intensity. They may also effectively treat sexual difficulties such as premature ejaculation, loss of interest, impotence, and difficulty achieving orgasm.

We do not propose a method of hyping up your sex drive with drugs at the expense of some other aspect of your health. Our orientation is more holistic. In fact, the new prosexual drugs and nutrients usually *improve* overall health. Many of the compounds discussed have a wide range of health benefits and have been shown in scientific studies to: enhance immune function, slow aging, alleviate depression, assist fat loss, improve memory, and more.

*Better Sex Through Chemistry* will be particularly useful for those of you who are healthy but just don't function as you once did (when you were, presumably, a wild, uncontrollable animal.) In other words, you have some degree of *age-related sexual decline*. This is where prosexual drugs and anti-aging medicine overlap, and is the most exciting material we cover.

*Better Sex Through Chemistry* will also be useful to those of you suffering from the negative sexual side effects of common prescription drugs (such as the antidepressants). Prozac, for instance, often causes some decrease in sex drive and interferes with the ability to achieve orgasm. There are some interesting possibilities for using prosexual drugs or nutrients to compensate for this side effect. You might also take a close look at the chapter on deprenyl, a prosexual drug that is also used to treat depression. (These issues should be discussed with your doctor.)

"Virtually all of the psychiatric medications I have worked with have sexual side effects."
— Martin Rubin, M.D.

*Better Sex Through Chemistry* is a practical and scientific book. We explain how each drug or nutrient works, how to use it, and how to obtain it, including detailed discussions of dosages, possible side effects, and precautions. We have also included many colorful stories of people who have used prosexual drugs to improve their sex lives and overall health.

## Sex and Overall Health

Sexual health is inseparable from overall health. If you improve your general state of health, you will invariably improve your sex function. In this book, we propose ways to improve your overall health and, in the process, enjoy the positive sexual "side effects."

We believe, however, that the connection between sex and health is a two-way street. In other words, enhancing sexual vitality and improving your sex life will also have a positive impact on your overall health. While we can't prove this proposition, there have been many individuals and cultures throughout history whose approach to health has reflected a similar point of view.

The ancient Chinese Taoists, for example, used an extensive array of herbal aphrodisiacs to increase sexual energy, believing that this practice would enhance overall health. In fact, the Taoists understood the flow of sexual energy within the human body as the very basis of physical and mental well-being. The intricate and exquisite Chinese *ars erotica* based on this principle were intended originally not to increase pleasure in sex, but to generate vitality for practitioners and extend lifespan. Channeling and modulating the flow of sexual energy was, in fact, believed to be the key to immortality. This belief in the primacy of sexual energy is expressed in the *yin/yang* symbol portraying the interplay of masculine and feminine forces as the fundamental principle of cosmic creation.

In Tantric Yoga, the locus of latent universal life-force in the human body is depicted as a snake coiled three times around a *lingam*, or phallus, at the base of the spine. Many schools of Yoga center their practice on the release and distribution of this energy, known as *kundalini*, for purposes of bodily purification and spiritual enlightenment. Tantrists view the kundalini as closely connected to sexuality. One of the ways it is activated and channeled is through ritualized sexual conjugation; and the culmination of the kundalini process is imaged as the union of a lover and her beloved.

> "The omnipresent process of sex, as it is woven into the whole texture of our man's or woman's body, is the pattern of all the process of our life."
> —Havelock Ellis

The renegade psychologist Wilhelm Reich viewed blockages to the free flow of sexual energy—which he called *orgone*—as the origin of neurosis. He eventually put forward the idea of orgone as a universal, pervasive cosmic energy.

All three of these schools of thought place sexuality at the very root of well-being; and to one degree or another, even at the root of being itself. And all of them suggest using sexuality as a starting point for improving overall health.

In conventional medical circles, sexual health is understood to be a key indicator of an individual's overall health. Some doctors ask patients about their sex lives (along with questions about sleep patterns, eating habits, etc.) when seeking a picture of their general condition.

The close relationship between sex function and other aspects of health is dramatically demonstrated by several of the prosexual drugs discussed in this book. For example:

→  Deprenyl is a prosexual drug. It also slows the progression of Parkinson's disease, enhances the mental acuity of Alzheimer's patients, extends the lifespans of laboratory animals, effectively combats depression, and more. How does it perform such a wide range of functions? By enhancing the activity of dopamine, a brain chemical that plays key roles in sex, aging, mood, cognition, and many other processes.

→  Bromocriptine is another prosexual drug. It can also help you lose weight. How? Largely by reducing levels of *prolactin* in the body. Prolactin naturally increases with age and is often to blame for age-associated impotence in men.

→  Gamma-hydroxybutyrate (GHB) is a prosexual drug for most people. It can also help you build muscle tissue, burn off fat, and sleep better. It works partly by triggering the release of growth hormone from the pituitary gland.

There are, incidentally, some drugs which may *temporarily* amplify certain aspects of sex function but are not particularly good for you in the long run. For example: amphetamine (speed) to increase sex drive, methaqualone (Quaaludes) to facilitate male erection, alcohol to release inhibitions, and MDMA (ecstasy) for intimacy and bonding. These substances may have their place, but would probably result in detriment to overall health—and therefore to sexual function—if used more than intermittently.

## Love Potions—Not!

Many readers will already have noticed that we have not referred to prosexual drugs as "aphrodisiacs." This decision reflects our desire to avoid the limitations and negative connotations of a term that we feel is largely obsolete.

Most dictionaries define an "aphrodisiac" as a substance or preparation that increases sexual desire. While most of the compounds discussed in this book can have this effect, this definition is far too limited to encompass the wide variety of effects and benefits that can be obtained from prosexual substances.

Furthermore, the word "aphrodisiac" is closely associated with the phrase "love potion." The latter term, which brings to mind images of witchcraft, magic, and foul-tasting brews, refers to a concoction which causes the person who ingests it to become sexually or romantically inclined towards the person who has prepared it. We know of no substances that can function in this manner.

## Our Research Methods

The research for this book included a large number of on-line searches of computerized medical databases for references to the "sex effects" of various drugs. In the process, we downloaded over ten megabytes in summaries of scientific papers—a volume of information that would fill about fifty books of this size. Additionally, we tracked down and read stacks of papers in full text, interviewed about 100 people for their personal anecdotes, and, of course, experimented on ourselves.

To our surprise, there is quite a bit more hard scientific data than we expected. Nevertheless, there are many substances that seem very promising in terms of prosexual properties that have not yet been fully explored in a scientific manner. Because we feel that our readers should know about these substances too, we have chosen not to base all of our entries in this book on purely scientific evidence. However, we feel strongly that readers should also know *what kind* of evidence is being used whenever a claim about a substance is made. We have therefore attempted throughout this book to state clearly the type of the evidence upon which all claims are based.

In deciding whether a substance was worthy of inclusion, we considered the following types of evidence:

### Controlled studies

The *double-blind, placebo-controlled trial* with human subjects is accepted by the scientific community as the most reliable and conclusive method for gathering information on the properties of drugs. Unfortunately, relatively few studies of this kind have been performed in the area of prosexual effects.

In this type of study (hereafter referred to as a *controlled study* for brevity), researchers attempt to control as many factors and conditions as possible that might effect the outcome of the experiment and the objectivity of the data gathered. This kind of study attempts to account for the well-known *placebo effect,* a phenomenon in which some subjects report a drug effect even though they have merely been given a dummy pill or injection—a placebo. In this scenario, the subject only believes they have been given the actual drug.

Double-blind studies divide experimental subjects into two groups: those receiving placebo, known as the *control group*; and those receiving the medication being tested. Consider the example of an experiment designed to test the efficacy of a substance in treating depression. A certain percentage of people suffering from clinical depression will improve without treatment over a given period of time. To the extent that the placebo effect applies to depression, a slightly greater percentage of subjects administered placebo will report signs of improvement. In order for a medication to be proven effective by the study, the percentage of subjects taking the drug that show improvement must be significantly greater than the percentage showing improvement in the control (placebo) group.

> "...interest in sex is very susceptible to the placebo effect."
> —Ward Dean, M.D.

Double-blind studies are devised to prevent psychological factors from affecting the way subjects report data and the way that researchers gather and document it. Neither the researchers conducting the experiment nor the patients themselves know which people are receiving placebo and which are receiving the substance being tested (hence the phrase "double-blind"). The placebo effect is thought to result from the patient's belief that he or she is taking a medicine that will have a particular effect, and would therefore not occur if the patient was *aware* that the substance was a placebo. Furthermore, the ignorance of the researchers prevents their prejudices and assumptions from biasing the information they report—for instance, tending to dismiss or overlook signs of improvement in the placebo group while exaggerating such signs in the group being administered "the real thing."

## Animal studies

In many cases scientific studies have been conducted which demonstrate the effects of certain substances on sexual behavior in animals. In the absence of equivalent human studies, there is no certainty that these substances will have similar effects in humans. Nonetheless, such evidence is sometimes strongly suggestive.

For example, Deprenyl, a relatively new drug gaining in popularity as a smart drug and life-extender, has been scientifically proven to have marked effects on the sex lives of rats. Deprenyl significantly increases the mounting frequency of middle-aged and older male rats (meaning that they have sex more often). Furthermore, rats given Deprenyl remain sexually active for a much longer portion of their lifespan, and the drug even revitalizes the

> "...anything that improves brain function is probably going to improve sexual functioning."
> —Ward Dean, M.D.

sex lives of older rats who had previously ceased to be sexually active. This scientific evidence for prosexual effects of Deprenyl derived from animal studies is accompanied by a large body of anecdotal evidence suggesting that the drug's sexual properties do in fact extend to humans; many corroborative reports have come from those who originally began using deprenyl for other purposes. Deprenyl is therefore a substance worthy of inclusion in this book in spite of the lack of scientific evidence regarding its sexual effects in humans.

## Anecdotal evidence

Anecdotal evidence consists of stories, reports, and personal testimonies. Such evidence can come from books, magazine articles, letters, journals documenting informal personal research, and verbal communications. The authors have also gathered a great deal of new anecdotal evidence in their research for this book by way of the numerous, often extensive personal interviews already mentioned. Some of the original impetus for this book came from the large number of anecdotal reports received in response to the smart drugs books concerning the beneficial sexual effects that readers had derived from many of the substances featured in those books.

### Informed speculation

Sometimes a substance has been proven to affect the physiological systems that underlie and support our sexual interests and capacities. For instance, a substance may increase the levels of one of the hormones involved in sexual attraction and arousal. Such evidence is strongly suggestive that the substance in question would have prosexual properties, but scientific studies conclusively demonstrating effects on sexual function and behavior may not yet have been performed. This category alone offers somewhat indirect evidence for prosexual effects, but can constitute part of a strong argument that the substance will be found to demonstrate such properties. When this kind of evidence is accompanied by strong evidence from another category—such as anecdotal evidence—we have chosen to include it in this book.

> "...the sexist bias in this research is clearly apparent, as pharmacological effects on female sexuality have been almost totally neglected by most investigators."
> —Rosen and Ashton
> *Prosexual Drugs...*

### An Example of How a Substance was Selected

Sometimes there is strong anecdotal evidence that a substance has prosexual value—and even a theoretical basis for understanding why or how it could function in this manner (informed speculation)—but no direct scientific confirmation. Such situations apply to many substances which seem to hold great promise as prosexual drugs.

For example, we have found no controlled studies investigating GHB for prosexual properties. However, those who have used GHB consistently report powerful prosexual results (anecdotal evidence). Additionally, we know from controlled studies that GHB boosts levels of *acetylcholine*, considered to be one of the body's natural prosexual chemicals. From this evidence we can infer that GHB is likely to have prosexual qualities (informed speculation). Taking into account all of these categories of evidence, we decided that GHB was clearly worth including.

### Other Considerations

Various factors in addition to the categories of evidence discussed above also played significant roles in our selection process. Those substances which appeared to be potentially beneficial to large numbers of people were favored over those which seemed likely to benefit only a relatively small group. Safety issues, of course, were of paramount importance: all of the compounds included feature extraordinarily high safety profiles. Other aspects of overall desirability were also taken into account. For instance, most men would no doubt prefer to take a few pills every day to enhance their erectile capacity than risk the eventual scarring of their genitals through long-term use of anti-impotence compounds that must be injected. (Several of these are currently being researched and publicized). Availability and legality were also important factors.

## The New Sexual Chemistry

By no means do we intend to address sex as if it were an exclusively biochemical issue. For many if not most people, love, intimacy, bonding, communication, tenderness, and even spirituality are essential for good sex. (It is not without reason that sex is called "making love," even when there is ostensibly no love involved.) We recognize that sex occurs in this broader context. We intend this book to be just as useful for people who find these elements important as for people who wish to concentrate their drive towards better sex in the somatic, sensory, hedonic dimension.

While we do not believe that sex is purely or exclusively biochemical, we do wish to emphasize that even the elements of sexuality that are usually thought of as non-physical do have a physical dimension. When this book deals with the more psycho-spiritual aspects of sex, it will do so mostly—but not exclusively—from the perspective of their largely neglected biochemical angle.

As science is clearly demonstrating, we can no longer ignore the biological aspects of the psychological and spiritual dimensions of human experience. For example, as a *Time* magazine cover story from early 1993 explains, scientists have made breakthroughs in understanding the biochemistry not just of sex, but of love and romance. And in the bestselling book *Listening to Prozac*, a prominent psychiatrist convincingly argues that this popular new "wonder drug" not only alleviates depression, but changes personality itself. This chemical is clearly acting as an effective biochemical agent of change in an arena of human existence previously relegated to the realm of the "purely" psychological.

As you will see, particularly in the case histories in this book, it is even possible to access and alter, biochemically, realms of sex such as intimacy, communication, and bonding.

While popular endeavors towards better sex have explored psychology, culture, and even spirituality, they have tended to ignore

"Look at Quaalude. Look at Ecstasy. When an illicit drug is a legitimate aphrodisiac, that's probably one of the reasons why it's illegal. Even though we have dozens of antidepressants because depression is a clinical condition classified as a disease, the FDA would be wary of drugs that take antidepressive action one step further and actually make you feel especially good. They disapprove of euphoriants."

—Ward Dean, M.D.

the inner workings of the body. This oversight, of course, has not been absolute. But even the exceptions tend to prove the rule: the ways in which physiology has been included in our search for better sex only reveal the extent of its general exclusion. Medical science has addressed sexual dysfunction with drugs and penile implants for male impotence, but its vast reserves of relevant information are usually forgotten when the goal becomes one of moving beyond the rudimentary competence of our sexual hardware towards a deeper level of sexual fulfillment. The "discovery" of the G-spot was perhaps most remarkable for the fact that this anatomical font of female pleasure had for so long been overlooked—and the professional debate as to whether it actually existed raged on even as untold numbers of women were already enthusiastically exploring its benefits!

It is clear, then, that biology and biochemistry have been at best unwelcome guests in our considerations of sex and romance. This is probably because science, at least in the eyes of most, is just not sexy, and certainly not romantic. When someone says something like, "love is just a chemical reaction" (hoping, perhaps, to put the pain of heartbreak into some sort of perspective), we usually consider him or her to be expressing a cold, cynical, and pessimistic viewpoint. The equation of love or sex with biology is thought to take the mystery, the romance, and the nobility out of sexuality, leaving lovers the hapless victims of inflexible, impersonal physical laws.

As it was put in the *Time* magazine article mentioned above, "most of us would just as soon not know" about the biological

"Human sexual behavior is extremely complex indeed. It has been described as the sum total of an individual's makeup, which includes chromosomal sex, gender identification, gonadal adequacy, rearing, environmental influences, hormonal factors, and possible hypothalamic sensitization."

—R.B. Greenblatt & A. Karpas
*Hormone therapy for sexual dysfunction*

underpinnings of our romantic and sexual lives. But even as we attempt to avoid the unavoidable, we implicitly acknowledge it in a myriad of ways. Recognition of the biochemical dimension of our sexuality is deeply embedded in colloquial vocabulary. When we ask a friend for a report on last night's first date, all he or she has to say is "no chemistry," and we nod sagely, knowing exactly what is meant: this first date will also be the last.

When it comes to an issue as important to us as our sex and love lives, we like to believe that we're in control. And if we can't convince ourselves that we are, apparently we'd prefer to believe at least that we're being buffeted about by mysterious spiritual or mystical forces that are more exciting and romantic than equations on a blackboard or the latest issue of *Scientific American.*

"Biology is destiny," reads a famous aphorism. When it is applied to sexuality, the truth that this quotation expresses has apparently been widely equated with pessimism. This reaction is based on the assumption that we're "stuck" with our biology—so if sex and love are in any fundamental way biological matters, there's little we can do to take charge of or improve these arenas of our lives. Such reasoning is no doubt the primary source of our tendency to deny the biochemical dimension of sex and romance. The *Time* article mentioned above perpetuates this point of view, stating that scientific knowledge of the biological underpinnings of love raises the "specter of determinism," implying that if our sex and love lives can be scientifically understood, somehow they can't be changed.

Nothing could be farther from the truth. Ironically, by refusing to consider, let alone embrace, the chemical element of love, we throw away the key to a sexual treasure chest whose inventory of potential gifts to our sexuality continues to expand as time passes.

These gifts to our sexuality are the new prosexual drugs. May they serve you well.

# Some Basic Physiology

The master gland of the endocrine system is the hypothalamus, located just beneath the brain near the top of the brain stem (approximately at the center of the head). It plays a central regulatory role in *homeostasis*, the maintenance (through various feedback systems) of the body's internal biochemical equilibrium in the face of changing external factors.

The anterior lobe, or forward portion, of the pituitary releases several hormones that play key roles in sexual and reproductive function, either directly or by stimulating other glands to release further hormones. For instance, this area of the pituitary secretes the hormones LH and FSH which, in men, regulate the testes and, in women, play roles in ovulation and the production of estrogen and progesterone. The anterior pituitary also releases ACTH which acts on the adrenals to stimulate the production of sex hormones. It secretes growth hormone, which appears to be a powerfully prosexual substance. The anterior pituitary also produces prolactin, a hormone which stimulates lactation in women. Prolactin has been implicated in the inhibition of sexual activity in lactating animals [Sodersten, 1983], and excessive levels are clearly associated with sexual dysfunction and decreased libido in men and sometimes women [Weizman, 1983].

The activities of the pituitary are regulated through the secretion of hormones by the hypothalamus, a part of the brain just above the pituitary at the top of the brain stem. The release of each pituitary hormone is under the influence of an opposing pair of hypothalamic hormones, one stimulating the release of the pituitary hormone and the other inhibiting it. Because the hypothalamus controls the pituitary, it is the locus "where the activity of the entire endocrine system is integrated." As such it is the organ most responsible for homeostasis. [Dilman, 1992].

The function of the hypothalamus, like all parts of the brain, relies on neurotransmitters, the "brain hormones" which transmit electrical messages or impulses from one brain cell to another. Some neurotransmitters important to hypothalamic function are dopamine, norepinephrine, serotonin, acetylcholine, histamine, gamma-amino butyric acid (GABA), and endorphins [Dilman, 1992].

In light of its controlling influence on the production of sex-related hormones by the pituitary and those glands in turn regulated by the pituitary, it is not surprising that within the hypothalamus has been located the brain's sex center. (In women, this actually consists of *two* sex centers: one regulating the surges of hormone production associated with the ovulatory cycle, and the other governing *basal* or ongoing levels of reproduction-related hormones.) The hypothalamic neurotransmitters most closely involved with the activity of the sex center are dopamine and norepinephrine, which charge its sex-related functions, and serotonin, which inhibits them.

Dopamine is widely equated with libido [Everitt, 1977] in both men and women, as is the hormone testosterone. In fact, hypothalamic dopamine plays an indirect role in stimulating testosterone production. It also inhibits pituitary secretion of prolactin, high levels of which may interfere with the production of testosterone's active form [Buffum, 1982]. As one journalist put it, in what is certainly an oversimplification, "For most people, there's a simple equation: more dopamine equals more libido" [Mellow-Whipkit, 1991]. Low dopamine levels have been linked with shyness, a finding with interesting implications for the relationship of this neurotransmitter to human socio-sexual interaction.

One process that has been found central to the phenomena of aging is the deterioration of the dopamine system, consisting of dopamine and those brain cells which release or respond to it. This decline is characterized by dwindling levels of dopamine, oxidative damage to neurons involved in dopamine transmission, and the corollary degeneration of the *substantia nigra*, the brain's primary center of dopamine manufacture. Considering dopamine's importance in stimulating the hypothalamic sex center, it makes sense that with aging (or with depression, a condition sometimes associated with low dopamine levels) often comes a decline in libido and sexual function.

The dopamine-sex connection thus takes place by way of the *hypothalamic-pituitary-gonadal axis*: the close relationship of the dopamine-fuelled hypothalamus with the pituitary, and the pituitary's regulation, in turn, of sex hormones and the glands that produce them. This connection accounts in large part for the success of bromocriptine and other dopamine agonists (substances that stimulate the dopamine system or increase levels of this neurotransmitter) in treating sex dysfunction related to aging and endocrine imbalances. It is also probably responsible for the prosexual reputation of some of these compounds, such as deprenyl, even among those with healthy libidos and no sexual "dysfunction" *per se*.

# Part I:

# Natural Substances

# Prosexual Nutrients

## *Prosexual uses of the nutrients:* ———————

**Men:** increased interest/desire; increased erectile capacity; increased stamina; ease of ejaculation; increased subjective enjoyment.

**Women:** increased interest/desire; increased frequency of orgasm; increased stamina and intensity of orgasm.

During the 19th century, a curious shift in attitude toward sexual behavior began to occur in the United States. The prevailing feeling at the time was that people who engaged in sex for reasons other than procreation were, quite simply, sinners and one day would find their true rewards in Hell. Starting in the early nineteenth century, however, a few apparently well-meaning people, who no doubt saw themselves as "enlightened," began to view masturbation and other forms of "excessive venery" not so much as sins as *medical* problems.

Of course, much of the medical wisdom they proffered was just as absurd and destructive as the religious attitudes, but at least it was a step in the right direction. Consider this piece of "medical" information from one Joseph W. Howe, MD, a professor of clinical surgery at Bellevue Hospital Medical College in New York City:

> *"The occurrence of seminal ejaculations three or four times a week from legitimate sexual congress will not be felt very much by a healthy man, while the same*

*number of losses from masturbation or nocturnal pollutions will soon superinduce mental and physical disability. Indeed there are many persons in robust health who indulge in daily intercourse with impunity, while others with perhaps equal stamina, lose flesh from two or three weekly pollutions. The reasons are obvious. One act is performed in accordance with the dictates of nature—the other is subversive and degrading"* [Howe, 1887].

Wouldn't you love to see the randomized, double-blind, controlled studies that led him to that conclusion!

While 19th century sexual attitudes moved away from condemning people to spiritual Hell, the medical alternative it offered may have been equally horrendous. Shame and damnation were replaced by fear of horrible diseases thought to arise from indulging one's sexual passions: blindness, epilepsy, impotence, sterility, insanity, vertigo, headache, physical weakness, loss of appetite, heart palpitations, insomnia, and so on.

Listening to these so-called sexual experts, one could easily gain the impression that sexual "excess" was the 19th century equivalent of the Black Death. For example, a self-appointed guardian of sexual health named Sylvester Graham wrote in 1834, "He who in any manner endeavors to excite the sexual appetites, and arouse the unchaste passions of youth, is one of the most heinous offenders against the welfare of mankind" [Graham, 1834].

It is useful to know that Graham wasn't talking about kiddie porn or child molesting here; he was talking about food. Along with other medical "experts" of the time, Graham believed in the power of prosexual nutrients, albeit as something to be avoided. Certain foods, he argued, were among the primary stimulants for sexual activity. He railed against "the free use of flesh," ie, eating a lot of meat, as well as the use of "stimulating seasonings and condiments, together with coffee, tea, rich pastry and compounded and concentrated forms of food; and too often, chewing and smoking tobacco, and drinking wine and other intoxicating liquors; all of which unduly stimulate and irritate the nervous system, heat the blood, and early develope [sic] a preternatural sensibility and prurience of the genital organs."

To prevent "the immense evils of self-pollution," Graham recommended that young people "subsist on a plain, simple, unstimulating, vegetable and water diet." Graham's legacy, of course, is still with us; it's called the Graham cracker.

Similar advice was offered by John Harvey Kellogg, MD, of Michigan, who suggested that concerned parents delay the development of puberty in their children by feeding them a diet consisting of oatmeal, Graham flour, ripe fruit, unbolted wheat flour, peas, beans, and other vegetables, which he said "are wholly free from injurious properties." Kellogg added that "a cool, unstimulating vegetable or farinaceous diet would deter the development of the sexual organism for several months, and perhaps for a year or two" [Kellogg, 1888].

People suffering from "sexual excesses," said Dr. Kellogg, should avoid all "stimulating" foods, such as spices, pepper, ginger, mustard, cinnamon, cloves, essences, all condiments, pickles, "flesh food in any but moderate quantities," chocolate, coffee, and tea.

## Prosexual Nutrients – 21st Century Style

While it's hard to imagine getting turned on by a jar of pickles, a hot dog smothered in mustard and spicy relish, or even a thick, juicy steak these days, scores of scientific studies and anecdotal reports suggest that certain nutrients can indeed contribute to sexual arousal, stamina, and satisfaction. For the most part, these nutrients, including the amino acids arginine, phenylalanine, and tyrosine, and the vitamins B-5, choline, and niacin all play important roles in facilitating and even enhancing neurotransmission and/or blood flow in regions of the brain and genital organs that control sexual function and sensation.

## L-Arginine and Sex: Just Say Yes to NO

Arginine is an essential amino acid, one of the building blocks of proteins in the body. "Essential" refers to the fact that the body cannot manufacture arginine from other substances the way it does with some (nonessential) amino acids. To maintain your supply of this nutrient, it is *essential* that you either consume foods containing arginine (eg, dairy products, nuts, chicken, turkey, and other fowl) or take L-arginine supplements.

Until about a decade ago, arginine was largely ignored except in its very limited protein-building role. Now it turns out, L-arginine is the main source of the primary molecule responsible for sexual arousal. It is interesting to note, however, that even back in the Dark Ages of the 19th century, people like Dr. Kellogg recognized the prosexual value of "nitrogenous elements of food," of which, it turns out, L-arginine is a major contributor.

The modern awakening to arginine use has come in three major waves. The first wave hit in the mid-1980s when Durk Pearson and Sandy Shaw popularized research showing that dietary L-arginine acts to release growth hormone (GH) from the pituitary gland at the base of the brain [Pearson, 1982; Merimee, 1969]. Injections of GH have since been shown to have dramatic anti-aging effects in older people, including increases in bone and muscle mass, decreases in fat, and improvements in skin tone [Rudman, 1990]. It seemed reasonable to assume that, since L-arginine induces a substantial natural release of GH [Knopf, 1965], it could have beneficial effects similar to those attributed to GH injections. The widespread successful use of supplements of L-arginine and other GH releasers by bodybuilders and other athletes testifies to the power of this amino acid.

A second wave of arginine research in the late 1980s demonstrated that L-arginine supplements significantly improve immune function [Barbul, 1990] and speed wound healing [Daley, 1988], also through the release of GH. Based on the remarkable recovery of seriously ill surgical patients taking arginine supplements, one prominent surgeon stated, "Arginine is an important dietary variable that could influence resistance to infection, especially those of the intracellular variety, as well as tumor growth and the development of metastasis" [Alexander, 1990].

### The primary mediator of penile erection

The third wave of arginine research hit in the early 1990s when scientists discovered that a simple gas known as nitric oxide (NO) may be one of the most important molecules in the body. You may have heard of NO's dark side. Just 10 years ago, it was thought of *only* as a toxic byproduct of automobile exhaust and other sources that pollute the atmosphere, cause acid rain, and destroy the ozone layer. Although NO is indeed dangerous in high concentrations, we now know that it plays a vital role in the normal function of the body.

Recent studies have confirmed that NO exercises considerable control over blood pressure, boosts immune function, kills cancer cells and microorganisms, and helps control muscular activity, balance, and coordination. Scientists also came to recognize NO as *the primary mediator of penile erection* [Burnett, 1992]. In 1992, *Science* magazine named NO its "Molecule of the Year." One researcher, in summarizing what is known about it in *The Lancet,* observed that "NO research is now riding on a crest of enthusiasm.... So far the basic research on NO has only just begun to make an impact on clinical medicine." [Anggard, 1994]. Another called work on NO one of the "hottest, most exciting things in neurobiology. Now a new kind of neurotransmitter turns out to be a gas. Good God!" [Hoffman, 1991].

What does NO have to do with sex and arginine? Quite simply, dietary arginine is the primary source of nitrogen molecules for NO. Without arginine in the diet, there would be no NO, and without NO there would be no erections. And, as will be seen below, arginine also plays a significant role in sexual function for women.

### Greater staying power and intensity

By facilitating blood flow to the erectile tissue of the penis, NO produced from L-arginine can give men erections that are bigger, harder, and more frequent. Some men also report that L-arginine gives them greater endurance. "It almost doubled my staying power," said one male enthusiast. Women also find it increases their "staying power." One highly athletic 30-something woman talked about the time she told her doctor about her L-arginine use. "My doctor almost fell off his chair when I told him how many times a night I do it—six times," she said. "He's definitely taking arginine now, too."

Because it helps increase the flow of blood to the penis, arginine can enhance erections. "I definitely have stiffer erections and more erections," said one man. "After I quit taking arginine for a while, I noticed that my hard-ons were not as big or as hard or as frequent," he added.

In women, L-arginine has been reported to increase the intensity of sensation during sex. "For me it's always been intense," said one long-time arginine fan, "but with arginine, it's even more intense."

### Enhanced libido

Both men and women have remarked about the way L-arginine seems to increase their libido, or desire for sex. Exclaimed one 21-year-old woman when asked about arginine, "My god, that stuff! I had to stop taking it. I was doing it with every guy that came along!" While her reaction may have been a bit extreme, some women have been reported to have given L-arginine to their husbands who had lost interest in sex and soon found a they had a rearoused mate on their hands.

### How does L-arginine work?

The prosexual effects of L-arginine are directly related to its ability to generate NO [Palmer, 1988]. NO molecules are produced on demand inside generator cells, such as the endothelial cells that line the insides of artery walls. An NO molecule is generated when an enzyme called *NO synthase (NOS)*, which is abundant in these cells, strips away a nitrogen atom (N) from a passing L-arginine molecule and combines it with an oxygen atom (O).

Since NO molecules have a very brief life span (their half-life is only about 5 seconds), their site of activity has to be very close to home. NO formed in arterial endothelial cells passes directly into immediately adjacent smooth muscle cells that surround the artery. This causes them to relax and leads to a reduction in blood pressure. A constant seepage of NO molecules is now identified as being crucial for controlling blood pressure [Anggard, 1994]. The more NO that is present, the lower the blood pressure, and vice versa.

When people have hypertension (high blood pressure) because their arterial endothelial cells are damaged and cannot make NO (a common finding in cardiovascular disease), their blood pressure drops after they receive an intravenous infusion of L-arginine [Drexler, 1991].

Dr. Salvador Moncada, research director at Wellcome Research Laboratories and a leading NO investigator, points out that if you place a drop of NO on the muscles that encircle a blood vessel, they instantly relax, which allows more blood to flow through them. He calls NO a "universal transducer," which is a kind of universal biochemical interpreter that translates chemical/electrical messages from one form to another [Kolata, 1991].

### The erection builder

Thanks to its relaxing effect on smooth muscle cells, NO is now widely recognized as the major, if not the sole neurochemical responsible for causing penile erections. Although acetylcholine (ACh) in the parasympathetic nerves that serve the penis has long been thought to be the major neurotransmitter involved in causing the penis to become erect, the most recent findings do not support this conclusion. ACh is certainly important for erections, but it is not the final step in the process. In laboratory experiments, blocking the cholinergic activity of these nerves does not necessarily affect the ability to have an erection. However, if you disrupt NO synthesis by applying chemicals that interfere with NOS activity, you completely prevent erections. NO synthesis can be restored after blocking NOS by supplying additional L-arginine [Burnett, 1992].

Dr. Arthur Burnett, a urologist at The Johns Hopkins University, and leading NO researcher, says that nitric oxide acts as an essential chemical trigger in producing erections. "It's like turning on a light switch." Noting that all you need to light up a room are wires, lamps and light bulbs, he adds, "It is the switch that starts the process." To light up your sexual life, it seems you need to flick the NO switch first [Associated Press, 1992].

To understand the role of NO in erections, it helps to understand how erections happen in the first place. Men get erections when sexual thoughts originating in the brain initiate a flow of nerve signals down the spinal cord to the arteries and smooth muscle in the penis. When they receive these signals, the arteries that supply the penis dilate and the muscles that control the two rods of sponge-like tissue filling the core of the penis—the corpora cavernosa and the corpus spongiosum—relax. As they relax, they allow the increased flow of blood through the penile arteries to fill the spongy space with blood. The increasing pressure in the penis compresses the veins that drain blood from the penis, preventing outflow. The more blood that fills the penis, the larger and harder the erection will be, because as long as blood is flowing in through the arteries, the outflow remains severely restricted. The penis returns to its flaccid state when the penile arteries constrict, relaxing pressure on the veins and allowing the blood to drain out. "We used to think that impotence was caused by poor inflow of blood to the penis," said Dr. Jacob Rajfer, a UCLA urologist. "We now know that most impotent men have a problem holding blood in the penis."

All these activities are under the control of NO molecules. The nerves that serve the spongy tissue and the penile arteries are, not surprisingly, rich in NOS. Thus, when you become sexually aroused, the NOS-rich nerves leap into action, kicking the conversion of L-arginine to NO into overdrive. The relatively large amounts of NO produced quickly diffuse to nearby arteries and smooth muscle, causing them to dilate and relax. NOS can be activated by a number of common substances released from nerves. Especially important is the neurotransmitter acetylcholine.

Penile erection has been studied in a variety of animal and *in vitro* (test tube) experiments. In one animal study, scientists injected one of three drugs into the corporal cavernosal tissue of primates. Two of the drugs, s-nitrocysteine (NO-CYS) and sodium nitroprusside (SNP), are direct sources of NO molecules. The third, acetylcholine (ACh), stimulates NOS to produce NO. For all three drugs, as the dose increased, so did the length, duration and hardness of the erections [Hellstrom, 1994]. Doing the same thing to cats gives a similar result [Wang, 1994].

Many people have experienced the prosexual effects of a NO-donating drug without even realizing it. The drug is amyl nitrate, which acts as a potent and short-acting vasodilator when inhaled. Many people inhale amyl nitrate just prior to sex. By rapidly lowering blood pressure, it can cause a momentary light headedness as well as a bigger, harder erection. In so doing, it can significantly intensify the experience.

## How does arginine work in women?

While anecdotal reports indicate that L-arginine has potent prosexual effects in both men and women, the actual mechanism of action in women is less clear. In female rats, NO release initiates a chain of events that begins with the pulsatile release of luteinizing hormone-releasing hormone (LHRH), followed by the release of LH, which leads to ovulation and also to behaviors like lordosis, which attract the male and facilitate mounting. Giving the rats a drug that inhibits production of NO, by blocking NOS activity, breaks this chain of behavior [Main, 1994].

Another rat study showed that NO produced in the rat uterus keeps the uterine muscle from contracting during pregnancy but not during delivery and that NO levels were controlled by the female hormone estrogen [Yallampalli, 1994]. In a result that would have warmed the hearts of Graham, Kellogg and their like, it has been found that completely depriving neonatal female rats of dietary arginine significantly slows their sexual development [Pau, 1982]. Perhaps, that's why they frowned on excessive meat eating. Meat is an excellent source of arginine.

## Can dietary L-arginine raise NO levels?

As long as your NOS system remains intact, it seems likely that additional supplies of L-arginine may increase the synthesis of NO. It is well-known that you can increase your brain levels of important neurotransmitters such as noradrenaline and acetylcholine by ingesting supplements of nutrients the body can use to make the neurotransmitters. Thus, it's also plausible that arginine supplements could increase the availability of NO.

### Why alcohol and sex don't mix

How many men have had the experience winding up in bed after a long night of drinking and found that nothing happened? They were impotent? It now appears that alcohol's well-known anti-sexual effects occur because it reduces the production of NO. In one recent study, researchers from the University of Pennsylvania took strips of rabbit corpus cavernosum tissue and bathed it in various solutions. They found that a solution of 5% alcohol significantly reduced the ability of the strips to relax when stimulated by a small electric current. When they added the drug nitroprusside, which supplies NO molecules, the muscle tissue behaved normally and relaxed when stimulated [Saito, 1994].

These data suggest that too much alcohol in the blood interrupts the normal production of NO, but they do not tell us at which step the interruption occurs. Does it block NOS activity? Does it affect L-arginine availability? Does it "eat up" NO molecules before they have chance to reach their destination? No one knows for sure. Thus, it's not known whether adding extra L-arginine to the system by taking a supplement should be able to overcome alcohol-induced inhibition of erection. Although it is certainly conceivable that L-arginine can improve sexual performance in people with this problem, we have had no anecdotal reports supporting this. If drinking interferes with your sexual activity, you might try taking some L-arginine before sex and see if it helps.

### Does L-arginine help impotence?

Drugs that *donate* NO molecules can cause an erection in impotent men. We have already mentioned nitroprusside and amyl nitrate. Unfortunately, powerful vasodilating drugs like these, which donate NO molecules, often have serious drawbacks. For example, to bring on an erection using papaverine, phentol-amine, or prostaglandin $E_1$, the drug must be injected into the base of the penis just before sex—hardly an appealing part foreplay. Another drug, glyceryl nitrate (*aka* nitroglycerine) can produce an erection when applied topically to the penis, but it has been known to give the man's sexual partner a headache! Not surprisingly, men who have tried these methods usually give them up pretty quickly.

According to Dr. Inigo Saenez de Tejada, chief of the urology laboratory at Boston University School of Medicine, the amount of NO produced in the penis is directly related to the magnitude of the erection. A lack of sufficient NO may be the reason men who smoke or have hypertension, atherosclerosis (clogged arteries), or diabetes become impotent so often. In fact, these are the major causes of physiologically based impotence. Blocked or damaged arteries are too narrow to permit sufficient blood-borne L-arginine and oxygen to reach the penis [Freundlich, 1993]. It is possible, at least in some men, that raising the concentration of L-arginine in the blood by ingesting supplements may help fill the nitrogen void. This possibility has not yet been studied systematically, however.

### Arginine and fertility

Anecdotal reports suggest that L-arginine supplements can improve fertility in men who have low sperm counts or poor sperm motility (activity). Durk Pearson and Sandy Shaw contend that L-arginine supplements can double sperm count in 2 weeks [Keller, 1975; Salvadorini, 1974]. In support, they tell the story of two male friends to whom they recommended L-arginine because sperm problems had prevented their wives from becoming pregnant.

> *"They were about to spend a lot of money on an attempt at in vitro fertilization. One month after starting on the arginine, the wives had both become pregnant! One of the men's doctors, surprised at the pregnancy, had asked for a sample of the man's sperm and, after examining it, accused our friend of giving him bull sperm, because, he said, the sample had too high a percentage of well-formed, motile sperm to be human sperm!"* [Pearson, 1991].

These conclusions are supported by research dating back to the late 1970s that show reduced levels of arginine in low quality human sperm [Papp, 1979]. Large animal breeders have known for decades that giving dietary arginine supplements to prize bulls and stallions enhances the animals' breeding potential. Arginine is also an important element of the diet in roosters used for breeding [Wilson, 1984].

### Side effects & adverse reactions

Published studies have indicated few serious problems related to taking L-arginine supplements. A few cautions about this amino acid are worth considering, however.

L-arginine may be problematic for some people with serious herpes infections. Once they enter the body, herpes viruses take up residence and generally remain dormant until stimulated into replication by factors such as stress or sunlight. Although L-arginine does nothing to initiate a herpes attack, once such an attack is stimulated, the virus may utilize the extra arginine molecules to enhance its replication, making the attack worse than it might have been otherwise [Griffith, 1981].

L-arginine should not be used if you have ocular or brain herpes. If you have any other problems with herpes, you should consult your physician before taking L-arginine [Pearson, 1986].

If you are diabetic or borderline diabetic, you should not use L-arginine or any GH-releaser, because it may make the disease worse by raising blood sugar levels. A few anecdotal reports also suggest that L-arginine may temporarily worsen arthritis in rare instances [Pearson, 1986].

GH-releasers do not produce cancer and have actually been shown to reduce the incidence of cancer in experimental animals. Nevertheless, if you have cancer, we recommend erring on the side of prudence and not taking L-arginine or any other GH-releaser because of the remote chance that the added GH may promote the growth of a pre-existing cancer.

Overall, it appears that high doses of L-arginine do not seem to cause serious problems. In the study of surgical healing mentioned earlier, "industrial strength" doses of arginine were given to very sick and debilitated people with no toxic effects [Daly, 1988]. Long-term use of high doses has not been studied, however.

As a final note, NO produced from L-arginine is a free radical. While free radicals are usually considered to be destructive and dangerous molecules that can alter DNA and wreak other cellular havoc in the body (antioxidant nutrients like vitamins C, E and beta-carotene are free radical scavengers), NO does not fit the standard free radical profile in some important ways. It has a very short life span (only a few seconds), which means it is neither as promiscuous nor as reactive as most other free radicals. In addition, because free radicals can only be destroyed by reacting with other free radicals, some scientists think that NO may be crucial for controlling other free radicals, since it reacts with them and neutralizes them before they can do any harm. In short, NO does not seem to have the destructive potential of typical free radical molecules, so you need not worry about creating extra free radicals when you take L-arginine.

### Dosage & timing

L-arginine users say they can achieve a prosexual effect by taking the amino acid supplement 45 minutes before sex. Pearson and Shaw recommend taking 6-18 grams of L-arginine in combination with 666-2000 milligrams of choline and about a third as much of vitamin B-5 (amounts dependent on sex and weight) one hour before vigorous exercise in order to facilitate the release of growth hormone from the pituitary. And they also point out that you can maximize the GH-releasing effect by avoiding eating any protein or other amino acid supplements (except for choline and phenylalanine) less than 3 hours before or 2 hours after taking the L-arginine. The reason is that these substances compete with arginine for the limited number of molecules available to transport amino acid molecules from the blood into the brain. It is not clear whether these guidelines are relevant if you are taking L-arginine just for sex.

Also, since most people take their arginine in a formulation that includes both choline and vitamin B-5, it is not known whether taking L-arginine by itself would have the same prosexual effects. Nevertheless, it seems that as long as you are going to the trouble to take L-arginine, why not take it with choline and vitamin B-5 and get the benefits of GH release too? As a bonus, the choline and vitamin B-5 may have prosexual benefits all their own. Choline is a major building block of ACh, which transmits impulses in the parasympathetic nerves that supply the genital area and ultimately release NO. Vitamin B-5 is required to produce Ach from choline and cholinergic drugs increase mucous membrane secretions. The two taken together may enhance sexual activity by increasing cholinergic nerve transmission leading to a greater than normal release of NO. (See the next section for more about choline and vitamin B-5.)

### *Availability and legal status*

L-arginine is legal and readily available as a nutritional supplement. It is sold as capsules, tablets, and powders in health food stores and by mail order. As mentioned above, it is often sold as part of a powdered formulation that also contains choline, vitamin B-5, and other nutrients, which can be mixed with water. Given the large amount that you need to take (up to 18 grams), the powdered formulation is easily the most convenient form.

## Choline and Vitamin B-5

Sexual arousal occurs not just in the genitals but in the whole body and, especially, in the brain. For men, it actually begins when the brain sends impulses down the spinal cord and out to the nerves that serve the penis. These impulses trigger the production of nitric oxide (NO), which causes penile arteries to dilate and the spongy core of the penis to relax and become engorged with blood. The neurotransmitter that carries the sexual message from the spinal nerves to the nerves that control the penile arteries and spongy tissue is acetylcholine (ACh). ACh also seems to control sexual behavior through its activity in the brain. For women, ACh is also a very important part of sexual function, as will be seen in the section below called "Evidence for cholinergic sexual effects."

Numerous studies confirm a key role for cholinergic nerve transmission in sexual responses. Simply speaking, with too little ACh, sexual activity goes down; increase ACh levels, and sexual activity goes up. Durk Pearson and Sandy Shaw have pointed out that ACh is involved in the build-up toward orgasm and the urethral and vaginal contractions that occur during orgasm as well as the subjective perception of orgasm intensity and duration [Pearson, 1984].

In addition to its direct role in the sexual response, ACh is also the primary chemical the body uses to transmit signals from nerves to skeletal muscles, the muscles that move the body. You need this chemical for muscular control and proper muscle tone. There is reason to believe that enhancing cholinergic neuromuscular transmission will enhance your energy and stamina by raising your ACh levels and that this can provide indirect sexual benefits by allowing you do it longer and with more energy.

While you can take drugs to enhance your body's cholinergic activity, these often have unpleasant or even dangerous side effects and are likely to be available only by prescription. One way to safely and effectively enhance your ACh levels is by taking supplements of choline, along with vitamin B-5, so that you body will manufacture more ACh.

### Evidence for cholinergic sexual effects

The results of several laboratory studies are beginning to draw a more detailed picture of the role of ACh in the sexual response. They reinforce the notion that female sexual responsiveness is controlled, at least in part, by ACh in the brain. When female rats were given the drug eserine, which increases brain levels of ACh, they exhibited the female receptive posture known as lordosis. When these same rats were then injected with the drug atropine, which blocks cholinergic transmission, the lordosis response to eserine vanished. The same thing happened when the anticholinergic drug scopolamine was infused into the rats' brains [Clemens, 1989]. In another experiment, the drug carbachol, which mimics the action of ACh, was injected into a region of the brain called the medial preoptic area and also stimulated lordosis [Clemens, 1981].

The role of ACh in the penis has been confirmed by studies in which strips of the spongy muscular core of human penile tissue are isolated in a bath containing noradrenaline, which causes it to contract. (In whole, living penises, noradrenergic stimulation contracts this muscle, leaving the penis flaccid.) When carbachol was added to the bath, the muscle relaxed.

Vitamin B-5, also known as pantothenic acid or calcium pantothenate, actually seems to enhance endurance by two routes. The first is its already-mentioned role in creating ACh from choline. Second, is its role in the energy-producing Krebs Cycle, which is vital for all living cells. An early indication that vitamin B-5 might increase physical endurance came from a study in which rats were placed into a tank filled with cool (64°F) water and forced to swim until they became exhausted. Prior to their swim, the rats' diets had included either high, adequate, or deficient levels of vitamin B-5. The high dose rats lasted more than four times as long as those whose diet had been B-5 deficient. In another experiment, pieces of frog muscle were stimulated electrically to make them twitch. The stimulation continued until the muscle became exhausted. Muscle tissue that was bathed in vitamin B-5 had double the work output as the control muscle. [Ralli, 1953].

### What are the sexual effects of choline and vitamin B-5?

As these results suggest, the primary sexual effect of treatment with choline and vitamin B-5 or B-5 alone is reported to be increased endurance. "I can generally have sex for about twice as long as I can without it," said a man in his 30s who takes vitamin B-5 by itself. "During cunnilingus, my tongue just doesn't get tired." One women, who uses choline plus vitamin B-5, says they help her feel more relaxed during sex. "There's no muscle tightness," she said. "It makes your body feel smoother, especially if you tend to tense up while having an orgasm."

### Dosage and timing

Experienced users recommend taking choline plus vitamin B-5 or B-5 by itself about 20 to 30 minutes before sex in order to get the full effect right from the start. But, notes one user, "Don't worry if you start too soon, it'll kick in as you're going." He adds that "Not everybody will notice it, but if you set a clock, you'll notice that you have the energy to go longer. Pretty much everyone I've told about B-5 has had that effect."

Many users take up to 3 grams of choline and up to 1 gram of vitamin B-5 (1/3 the amount of choline) each day when taking L-arginine as a GH releaser. It is common for people who want to enhance their sexual endurance to take at least half their dose prior to sex. It is probably advisable to begin with a lower dosage (perhaps 1 gram of choline and 1/3 gram vitamin B-5 per day) and to increase the dose over a period of several days to avoid any side effects.

### Side effects & adverse reactions

Because increasing ACh levels increases muscle tone, taking too much can cause a muscle tension headache or stiff, tight muscles, especially in the neck and shoulders. Also, taking high doses of choline and vitamin B-5 too soon can give you intestinal cramps as the ACh stimulates your gut muscles. Since this stimulation can speed food through your intestinal tract, high doses may give you anything from a mild laxative effect to diarrhea. If this happens, you can skip the nutrients for 1 or 2 days and then reduce the dose by half before gradually increasing it again. Many people have noticed that tolerance to the muscle tone-increasing effect develops quickly.

### Legality and availability

Both choline and vitamin B-5 are legal and are sold in health food stores and by mail order in capsules and powders by themselves and as part of various formulations. The FDA recognizes both choline and B-5 as nutrients, but has not approved them as agents for enhancing sexuality, improving muscle tone, speeding intestinal peristalsis, or as an adjunct to arginine in GH release.

## Niacin

Anyone who has taken megadoses of vitamins has probably experienced a niacin flush. Your skin gets warm and red and itchy and stays that way for 10 to 20 minutes. If you are not expecting it and do not know what it is, a niacin flush can be alarming and some people find the feeling uncomfortable. In fact, a niacin flush is quite harmless and can be used to great advantage as a means of increasing your sexual pleasure.

### Enhancing the natural "sex flush"

The flush occurs when niacin (also known as vitamin B-3 or nicotinic acid) causes a large release of histamine all over the body, one effect of which is to dilate blood vessels so more blood can flow through them. A relatively large release of histamine occurs naturally during sexual excitation and is thought to cause a "sex flush" in the face, neck, shoulders, chest, and other areas. This has been documented by Masters and Johnson. The flush caused by niacin is basically the same as the natural "sex flush" but is probably more intense. The niacin-induced histamine release also causes secretion of mucus in the mouth and sexual organs, enhancing that normally produced in response to sexual activity.

People who use niacin prior to sex remark about its ability to increase sensation, and not just in the genital area. Skin-to-skin contact all over the body during a niacin flush can be extraordinary. Because it is so safe and inexpensive, niacin is a very popular prosexual nutrient. Exclaimed one satisfied user, when asked about niacin, "Everybody knows about that. It's well-known up and down Main Street in Santa Monica. You take some before sex and WOW!"

Niacin may also help some people who have trouble achieving orgasm, since an adequate release of histamine is required to experience an orgasm. Pearson and Shaw tell the story of a thoroughbred stallion that could not reach orgasm until they recommended giving it niacin supplements. The strategy worked beyond their wildest dreams. "In fact," they wrote, "[the handlers] even had to restrain the horse because they were afraid he might injure himself by the frequent masturbation in which the stallion then engaged!" [Pearson, 1982].

### Side effects & adverse reactions

Ironically, the niacin flush is usually considered to be a side effect of this nutrient. It is dose-dependent, and if you regularly take high doses, you will find that you quickly develop tolerance to it. Pearson and Shaw remarked that one of the best ways they have found for helping people to become accustomed to the niacin flush is to try using it before sex [Pearson, 1982].

Since niacin is a fairly strong acid (nicotinic acid), high doses can cause acid indigestion. It can also contribute to acid indigestion by causing a release of histamine in the stomach, which leads to the release of even more acid. You can counter this by taking a formulation of niacin that has been buffered with a magnesium salt or by taking an antacid along with the niacin. Be careful though, because too much magnesium can give you diarrhea.

It is generally recommended that if you take individual doses of niacin over 200 milligrams or daily doses higher than 800 milligrams, that you do so under the supervision of your doctor, because high doses can occasionally cause liver malfunction. A simple blood test will detect any abnormality and lowering the dose will quickly eliminate the problem. Diabetics, people with active ulcers, and people being treated with certain drugs for tuberculosis should also refrain from using high doses of niacin unless their doctor approves.

### Dosage and timing

The dose of niacin you require to cause a flush varies depending on your sensitivity. If you do not take niacin regularly, you may be able to induce a good flush with as little as 50 milligrams. But if you have been taking megadoses of niacin for its nutrition benefits, you have probably already built up a tolerance to flushing and will have to increase your dose significantly.

It is best to take the niacin on an empty stomach, a practice that is usually discouraged because it increases the chances of a flush. Another way is to stop taking the niacin for a couple of days. You will lose some tolerance, and your regular dose may then give you a flush. Be sure to avoid taking a time-release niacin formulation or niacinamide, another form of vitamin B-3. These are specifically designed to avoid the flush.

Users find that the flush occurs about 15 to 30 minutes after ingesting the niacin and lasts from 10 to 20 minutes. For best results, you may want to be at peak flush when you reach orgasm. You will probably have to experiment to find the dose and timing that is right for you.

## Tyrosine and Phenylalanine

Several lines of evidence link activity of the neurotransmitter dopamine in the brain with sexual behavior (see the chapter called "Some Basic Physiology.") Generally, it appears that higher levels of dopamine are associated with more sexual interest and vice versa. Increased brain dopamine activity caused by taking the drug L-dopa is believed to be the cause of a "hypersexuality" syndrome in people who take the drug for Parkinson's disease.

L-dopa is a chemical precursor of dopamine (which in turn is a precursor of norepinephrine). In other words, the body uses L-dopa to make dopamine. L-dopa is available only by prescription, but you can also increase your brain dopamine levels by taking the nonprescription amino acids that the body uses to make L-dopa: tyrosine and phenylalanine (see diagram on page ?).

People who have lost interest in sex because they are depressed may benefit from taking doses of 100 to 500 milligrams of L-phenylalanine or L-tyrosine for 2 weeks. Supplements of vitamin B-6, vitamin C, folic acid, and copper in addition to the tyrosine or phenylalanine, should help maximize the conversion of L-dopa to dopamine [Pearson, 1982, 1984, 1991].

### Safety and adverse effects

High doses of phenylalanine or tyrosine can increase blood pressure in a few sensitive people who already have hypertension. It is best to start out at a low dose and increase the dose slowly over several days to several weeks, while keeping a close watch on your blood pressure. People who are taking a type of antidepressant drug known as a monoamine oxidase inhibitor (or MAO inhibitor or MAOI) should not take these amino acids, since the combination could cause a hazardous rise in blood pressure. Deprenyl (see the chapter on Deprenyl) may be an exception to this rule.

### Legality and availability

Supplements of L-phenylalanine and L-tyrosine are legal and readily available in health food stores and by mail order.

## Physicians and Product Sources

Please note the tearout card at the front of this book where you will find instructions for getting our *Directory of Mail Order Pharmacies* and *Directory of Physicians*. These listings are updated monthly. (Please also read the 'Disclaimer' section at the front of this book.)

*"I discovered GHB at a time when my sex life had no more life to it. I was stressed out, feeling unattractive, losing interest in sex, and my erections were a bit difficult to hold. GHB changed all that. It vastly enhanced my libido and I was harder for longer. In bed I felt wild and renewed."*

—30-year-old man

# GHB

## Prosexual uses of GHB: _____

| | |
|---|---|
| **Men:** | ease of erection; stability of erection; postponement of ejaculation. |
| **Women:** | greater intensity of orgasm; increase in vaginal sensitivity. |
| **Men & Women:** | disinhibition; increased interest in sex; increased tactility; increased bonding; emotional intensity; intimacy. |

GHB, or gamma-hydroxybutyrate, is a normal constituent of mammalian biochemistry. It is found naturally in every cell in the human body. In the brain, the highest amounts occur in the hypothalamus and basal ganglia [Gallimberti, 1989]. GHB is found in even greater concentrations in the kidney, heart, skeletal muscles, and brown fat [Chin, 1992]. It is believed to be a neurotransmitter, although the jury is still out as to whether it exhibits all of the properties required for fulfillment of this function [Chin, 1992]. It is both a metabolite and precursor of the inhibitory neurotransmitter GABA (gamma-aminobutyric acid), to which it bears a close relationship of chemical structure. GHB, however, does not act on GABA receptor sites [Chin, 1992].

GHB was first synthesized about thirty years ago by H. Laborit, a French researcher interested in exploring the effects of

GABA in the brain. Direct administration of GABA would not be effective for this purpose because it does not cross the blood-brain barrier. Laborit's alternative was to administer GHB, which *does* cross the blood-brain barrier, and some of which, once inside the brain, metabolizes into GABA [Vickers, 1969].

Independently of its relationship to GABA, however, GHB turned out to be a drug with its own range of effects. It has since been widely used and researched, finding applications in obstetrics and general anesthesia and in the treatment of alcohol withdrawal syndrome, narcolepsy, insomnia, and other arenas.

During the 1980s, GHB was widely available over-the-counter in health-food stores, purchased largely by body-builders for its ability to aid in fat reduction and muscle-building. In the last few years it has been gaining popularity as a "recreational" drug offering

One pleasantly surprised man earned the title of "angel" merely by sharing some GHB with two of his friends. After having been hosted on an out-of town trip by a married couple in their forties, as a parting gift he left them with some GHB and instructions for use.

A few weeks later, they phoned him, overflowing with gratitude. They revealed that, prior to visitation by their GHB "angel," as they called him, their marriage had been headed towards divorce; their sex life had fizzled out; and they had been spiralling into alcoholism.

After a few sessions using GHB together, their relationship had turned around. Barriers to communication that had become seemingly impenetrable had dissolved under the disinhibiting effects of the drug; their sex life had been re-ignited by its aphrodisiac properties; and their desire for alcohol—a substance they found considerably less attractive by comparison to GHB—had completely evaporated.

A marriage on the rocks had been granted new life by a series of crucial breakthroughs—each of them catalyzed, the couple agreed, by GHB.

a pleasant, alcohol-like, hangover-free "high" and potent prosexual effects.

## The Demonization of GHB

A long-lived media truism holds that "all publicity is good publicity." The recent history of GHB might serve as a case in point.

Most of those who've heard of GHB probably first became aware of it by way of a widespread rumor—unsupported by the subsequent coroner's report—that it played a role in the death of actor River Phoenix in the Fall of 1993. An article in the December 6th issue of *Newsweek* reported that this piece of hearsay—despite its alarming nature—inspired a groundswell of demand for GHB in the nightclub drug underground. Newsweek reported: "The hunt was on. *'I'd never heard of GHB before. No one in New York had,'* said a Manhattan drug user. *'This month it's the only drug'*" [Rogers, 1993].

The facts were widely misrepresented in the popular media, which vastly exaggerated GHB's so-called "dangers"— and usually left them unspecified. For instance, *Newsweek* sensationally described GHB as "an obscure and dangerous steroid substitute occasionally gulped down by West Coast thrillseekers" [Rogers, 1993]. (Although it can be used to increase muscle mass, GHB is neither a "steroid" nor in any other way "steroid-like," as it was often rendered in even more distorted reports.) And a guide to aphrodisiacs published in 1993 made a vague reference to "dangerous side effects" in the first sentence of its description of the drug [Watson, 1993].

In 1992, a report written by epidemiologist Ming-Yan Chin and Richard A. Kreutzer, MD, both staff members of the California Department of Health Services, warned sternly of GHB's "tremendous potential for abuse." Nonetheless, the authors went on to conclude: "there are no documented reports of long term [detrimental] effects. Nor is there any evidence for physiologic addiction." (See "Addictive potential" in the "Safety Issues" section.) [Chin, 1992.]

What, then, was the source of their concern? By way of

explanation for "sounding the alarm," Chin and Kreutzer offered only the following statement: "All interviewed patients reported a pleasurable sensation or a 'high.' Several of them explicitly noted that one reason they continued taking the drug was because it made them 'feel good.'" It would seem that the authors construed "feeling good"—in and of itself—as a threat to the public health in whose service they were ostensibly employed.

For whatever reasons, the FDA banned the over-the-counter sale of GHB on November 8th, 1990 [Chin, 1992].

## Setting the Record Straight

More than twenty-five years of scientific research into the effects of GHB—right up to 1989, one year prior to the FDA ban—clearly contradicts GHB's U.S. media image as a menacing poison. It will become clear as this chapter unfolds that numerous beneficial physiological effects—in the absence of significant negative physiological consequences—are well-documented in the scientific literature. Additionally, there is strong anecdotal evidence for psychological and sexual benefits.

In fact, prior to the FDA ban, GHB's high degree of safety was practically taken for granted in the scientific literature. A 1964 report lists "very low toxicity" as one of the "principle elements" of the GHB's pharmacology [Laborit, 1964]. A 1969 summary of its anesthetic uses called GHB "a truly nontoxic hypnotic," repeatedly emphasized its "lack of toxicity," and cited evidence that it demonstrates "no toxic effects on the liver and kidney" [Vickers, 1969]. In describing the way GHB is metabolized, a 1972 paper mentions "the absence of any need of detoxication by the organism" [Laborit, 1972].

As recently as 1989, this scientific picture of GHB's benign nature remained unchanged. A study from that year on its uses in treating alcohol withdrawal in humans notes that "GHB action...seems to be without serious side effects." The same report's almost off-hand reference to the "safety of GHB" shows how well-established this property of the drug had become [Gallimberti, 1989].

### Worst-case scenarios

Chin and Kreutzer's 1992 document, summarizing ten cases of "Acute poisonings associated with gammahydroxybutyrate in California," thus represented a radical departure from the previous consensus. (It is worth noting that "poisoning" was never defined in this paper.) Four of the cases reported involved "unknown doses." Four featured the "coingestion" of other drugs, usually alcohol. One involved unmedicated epilepsy and another a history of *grand mal* seizures—conditions specifically contraindicated for GHB. Chin and Kreutzer acknowledged that the "more severe reactions... generally occurred when patients took an unmeasured dose, a particularly large dose, or several doses within a short period of time."

The two most severe incidents of adverse reaction out of the ten included in Chin and Kreutzer's document are by far the most extreme cases encountered in the wide-ranging research on GHB performed for this book. Both of these cases involved the ingestion of central nervous system depressants in addition to GHB.

"Even the FDA," says physician Ward Dean, "admits that there have been no deaths attributable to this drug."

(Combining GHB with central nervous system depressants, such as alcohol or tranquilizers, is generally considered inadvisable.) They are included here as "worst case scenarios" to guarantee that the complete spectrum of GHB's potential effects is represented.

One of Chin and Kreutzer's case histories relates the story of a "previously healthy 39-year old Caucasian woman." During the period of her experimentation with GHB, she was also using Vicodin, a prescription painkiller containing a central nervous system depressant. She "experienced numbing of the legs, dizziness, and a tight chest" after her first dose of GHB (consisting of one teaspoon) purchased from a health-food store. Nonetheless, this woman resumed taking GHB three weeks later. For one month thereafter, she took one-half teaspoon of GHB on a near-daily basis without negative consequence.

However, after the last of "three or four doses" consumed on a day during which she departed from this regimen, "she experienced a 'high'...the 'jabbers' (pressured speech and ebullience), intense drowsiness, confusion, trouble breathing, and uncontrollable twitching in her arm. Her children found her and reported that her eyes were rolled back, her body was tense, and"—although no mention is made as to how the children were able to make such a determination—"she was hallucinating."

She was admitted to a hospital for a night, where, despite the disturbing nature of the symptoms recounted above, it was determined that "her pulse, blood pressure, and respiration were normal." Her physical exam was deemed "unremarkable except for alternating wakeful and sleepy states with irregular leg twitches."

> In all of the cases of "poisonings" reported by Chin and Kreutzer, rapid and spontaneous recovery occurred without treatment, usually within a matter of hours, and was followed by no further symptoms.

Her case history concludes: "she experienced a full recovery with no lasting symptoms."

The second case involves a "28-year old Caucasian woman" who took an unspecified quantity of GHB in addition to "some mixed drinks" at a nightclub. The report continues: "she experienced confusion and uncontrollable shaking followed by a seizure and then coma. A witness states that she was banging her head on a wall before becoming unconscious. Patient vomited and was suctioned before transport. Paramedics reported that she alternated between combativeness and unresponsiveness as she was taken to the emergency room. She arrived...with good respiratory effort but with long apneic periods [lapses of breathing]." Her recovery was complete, with "no adverse side effects" since the incident.

Several points regarding this case are worth keeping in mind. The woman's blood alcohol level was assessed at the hospital and was found to be quite high. Furthermore, it seems likely from the context of Chin and Kreutzer's presentation that the GHB may have been acquired at the nightclub where the incident took place. Under such circumstances, and in light of the severity of the woman's reaction, the possibility must be taken into account that the substance in question may in fact *not* have been GHB at all. Lastly, the report of "seizure and then coma" need not be the great cause for alarm that it at first seems—as will be explained shortly. (And in any case, this woman's "coma" must have been rather short-lived in order for her to be able to behave in a "combative" manner towards paramedics.)

Another of Chin and Kreutzer's cases is worthy of mention not for its *severity* but for its *mildness*. In this incident, a "39-year-old Caucasian man" took a rather large quantity of GHB (one and a half teaspoons, or nearly four grams) along with twenty-five milligrams of diphenhydramine hydrochloride (another central nervous system depressant, marketed over-the-counter both for allergies and as an aid to sleep). The *only* reported symptom is that he became "lethargic." This effect hardly seems disturbing given that he had just taken two known hypnotics (although it apparently disturbed his wife, who called 911 and had him taken to an emergency room—from which he was released in two hours). It is especially difficult to understand why this case is included among so-called "poisonings."

Despite their alarmist tone, the authors acknowledge that "there have not been any reported deaths" and that "if product use is discontinued, full recovery with no long-term side effects is universal." They concluded that "the prognosis for people who experience GHB poisoning is quite good."

Summarizing the results of Canadian research into GHB as a treatment for narcolepsy, authors Chin and Kreutzer further undermine their own stated position on GHB's abuse potential by reporting that:

> *"Several researchers...consistently describe the beneficial clinical effects...One Canadian researcher has noted adverse effects no worse than abrupt sedation, ataxia [lack of coordination], sleepwalking, unarousability, and decreased inhibition in normals [meaning persons free of narcolepsy or other major disease conditions] taking two to six teaspoons twice a night for several years. One patient who accidentally*

*took fifteen teaspoons on one occasion suffered no adverse reactions other than deep sedation and a headache the next day. No investigator reported any long-term adverse effects, addictive or dependent qualities associated with discontinued usage of the drug."* (See "Addictive potential" in the Safety section.)

Chin and Kreutzer acknowledge that "Researchers working with narcoleptics consider GHB a relatively harmless and effective drug" [Chin, 1992].

### *"Comas and Seizures" or "Sleeping and Twitching"?*

Negative press on GHB frequently mentions the possibility of "seizures" and "coma." These are certainly frightening words—until their meaning is closely examined in context.

With regard to GHB, "coma" refers merely to the state of deep sleep or unconsciousness induced by higher doses, from which people often cannot be aroused until the GHB has worn off. This "coma" is of short duration—one to two hours—and provides the basis for GHB's use as a general anesthetic. In fact, one researcher even described it as a "nontoxic coma," [Vickers, 1969] a phrase that in itself defuses much of the fear inspired by the use of the word.

This state of "coma" could just as easily—and accurately—be described as one of "unarousability" (the key term in the definition of "coma") or "deep sedation." In fact, these are the words used by Chin and Kreutzer themselves in their summary of research results from Canada, quoted above.

Their phrases "adverse effects no worse than...unarousability" and "no adverse reactions other than deep sedation" would have quite a different impact if the word "coma" was inserted in place of its synonyms. In fact, the alternate phrases created thereby—"adverse effects no worse than...*coma*" and "no adverse reactions other than *coma*"—appear blatantly self-contradictory. Nevertheless, there is no significant difference here in *meaning*, only in choice of *terminology*.

The point here is that the wording chosen by the major media and other sources in public discourse about GHB has carried a substantial negative load.

Like "coma," the word "seizure" becomes much less frightening when it is replaced by alternatives that are considerably less "loaded" but nonetheless equally accurate in terms of GHB's actual observed side effects. The "seizures" sometimes associated with GHB are usually described as being of the "clonic" variety [Vickers, 1969; Chin, 1992]. This word refers to "a forced series of alternating contractions and partial relaxations of a muscle" [Webster's 7th New Collegiate], as in one researcher's statement that "During the onset of [GHB] coma...random clonic movements of the limbs or face are frequently seen." This activity could alternatively—and correctly—be described as "muscle spasms" or "twitching."

Thus, a dire-sounding warning such as "a large dose of GHB can cause coma and seizures" could be translated into the relatively innocuous statement that "a sufficient dose of GHB may result in a few hours of deep sleep from which the user cannot be aroused, and the entry into unconsciousness may be accompanied by some twitching of the face or limbs."

## Why Was GHB Banned?

It seems likely, then, that at least some of the motives behind the 1990 FDA ban of GHB were other than those of public safety. Such a ban constitutes the only means of Federal control of a drug neither scheduled by the DEA nor approved by the FDA for prescription use. (The latter status requires considerable expenditure

"Dr. Cotzias, the inventor of L-dopa therapy for Parkinsonism, personally told us that the FDA delayed approval of L-DOPA for years because of its aphrodisiac side effects, and that aphrodisiac side effects are a greater block to FDA approval than carcinogenic side effects!"

—Pearson & Shaw [1988]

of time and money on the part of a pharmaceutical firm in an investment that can usually be recovered only when the company in question holds an exclusive U.S. patent. In the case of GHB, no such patent exists.) As physician Ward Dean has put it, "the FDA doesn't like drugs that people use just to 'feel good' or unwind after a hard day's work. In fact, the aphrodisiac properties of GHB may well have been part of the motivation for the ban" [Dean, 1993].

## What Are the Real Concerns?

The purpose of this section has been to make clear that the dangers widely attributed to GHB have been greatly exaggerated. Were this not the case—and were not the benefits offered by GHB both substantive and well-documented—a drug so controversial, and so ambiguous in legal status, would not have been included in this book. Such an argument having been made, it must be emphasized that, as with most substances, unpleasant—although not ultimately dangerous—side effects *can* be associated with GHB. Furthermore, there is one potentially significant hazard that must be taken into account when self-administering GHB: a sufficient dose—usually only about twice the amount required for a pleasant prosexual effect—can, as one user put it, "knock you out, but *fast*." (To keep things in perspective, remember that alcohol—a drug of exponentially greater toxicity and health risk than GHB—and many approved prescription drugs can also function in this manner.)

Durk Pearson and Sandy Shaw's book *Life Extension: A Practical Scientific Approach* features a chapter entitled "Is There Anything Perfectly Safe?" The entire text of this chapter consists of a single capitalized word: "NO" [Pearson & Shaw, 1982]. This succinct statement applies to GHB. In spite of its general safety and lack of toxicity, the intelligent use of GHB requires preparation, information, care, caution, and good judgement. These issues will be fully discussed in the sections called "Safety Issues" and "Self-Administration."

## How Does It Feel?

Most users find the "high" induced by GHB to be a pleasant state of relaxation and tranquility. Many compare it to the state afforded by alcohol; others mention "Quaaludes," minor tranquilizers such as Valium or Xanax, or marijuana. Others draw parallels with their experiences in meditation or following sessions of deep massage. Those who experience emotional release, heart-opening qualities, and facilitation of intimate verbal communication are sometimes reminded of MDMA ("Ecstasy").

The morning after effects of GHB lack the unpleasant or debilitating characteristics associated with some of these other drugs. In fact, many users report feeling particularly refreshed, even energized, the next day. As one woman put it, "I look at it as like being really high on alcohol, without the body poisoning."

The effects of GHB can generally be felt within five to twenty minutes after ingestion. They usually last no more than one and a half to three hours—although they can be indefinitely prolonged through repeated dosing. Placidity, sensuality, mild euphoria, and a tendency to verbalize often characterize the "high." Anxieties and inhibitions tend to dissolve into a feeling of emotional warmth, well-being, and pleasant drowsiness. A forty-one year old female singer-songwriter describes the GHB state in terms of "...a certain sensual, very blissful quality. It also gives you reduced inhibitions."

The effects of GHB are very dose-dependent. This means that small increases in the amount ingested lead to significant intensification of the effect. Higher levels feature greater giddiness, silliness, interference with mobility and verbal coherence, and sometimes dizziness. Doses slightly higher than those required for such effects will usually induce sleep.

The nature of the GHB "high" will be further discussed in the section entitled "GHB and Sex." Control and modulation of the "high," and its relationship to dosage, will be further elaborated in the section on "Self-Administration." Unpleasant sensations and effects that can sometimes arise will be discussed under "Precautions, Side Effects, and Contraindications."

## The Action of GHB in the Body

GHB significantly alters concentrations of the neurotransmitter dopamine and levels of two hormones released by the pituitary gland: growth hormone and prolactin. It also features several other benign metabolic, biochemical, and physiological effects.

### Dopamine

GHB can double concentrations of dopamine in the brain. This dopamine increase is specific to certain brain regions [Laborit, 1972], including the *substantia nigra,* a major center of dopamine manufacture [Chin, 1992]. (For more information on dopamine and its functions, see the chapters "Bromocriptine" and "Some Basic Physiology.") It is possible to inhibit this effect with other substances, including naloxone, caffeine, and amphetamines [Chin, 1992].

Oddly enough, this heightening of brain dopamine levels does not, at least initially, lead to increased activity of the brain's dopamine system. Rather, GHB increases dopamine concentrations by *inhibiting* the release of dopamine from nerve endings. This creates higher levels of the neurotransmitter within the brain cells where it is stored.

Some scientists have speculated that this buildup of dopamine may be released into the synapses after GHB wears off [Chin, 1992]. This could lead to feelings of increased well-being, alertness, and arousal associated with greater dopamine activity the next day.

### Growth hormone

GHB is a potent stimulator of the release of growth hormone by the pituitary. One article notes that the "increased GH [growth hormone] secretion produced by GHB administration is far in excess of any other previously available GH stimulator" [Fowkes, 1993]. As discussed in the chapter on bromocriptine, growth hormone, which stimulates the body to burn its own fat for fuel and to grow new muscle tissue, is attributed with life-extending, immune-enhancing, and prosexual effects.

One Japanese study reported in 1977 involved six healthy men between the ages of twenty-five and forty. Blood levels of growth hormone were tracked across a period of two hours after intravenous injection of 2.5 grams of GHB, and compared to control or baseline levels assayed in the same men across a similar period of time after injection of placebo (saline solution). Growth hormone levels increased by a factor of nine within thirty minutes, and peaked at

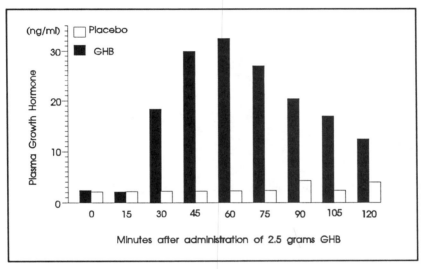

sixty minutes at a level *sixteen times* that of baseline. Thereafter, growth hormone levels began to decline gradually, but were still seven to eight times higher than normal at the two-hour point [Takahara, 1977].

The mechanism by which GHB stimulates growth-hormone release is not known. As described in the chapters "Some Basic Physiology" and "Bromocriptine," dopamine activity in the hypothalamus stimulates pituitary release of growth hormone. Thus, many dopaminergic drugs function as growth-hormone releasers. However, as has been noted, GHB actually *inhibits* the release of dopamine from nerve terminals, leaving its growth hormone stimulating effects—which must take place through an entirely different route—something of a mystery [Takahara, 1977].

### Prolactin

The same Japanese study discussed above also assayed the response of blood prolactin levels to GHB injection. Serum prolactin levels increased along a curve contoured similarly to that for growth hormone, peaking at the sixty-minute point at a level more than five times greater than baseline [Takahara, 1977]. This effect, unlike the release of growth hormone, is entirely consistent with GHB's inhibition of dopamine. Other compounds which dampen dopamine activity in the brain, such as the neuroleptic Thorazine, have been shown to result in pituitary prolactin release.

GHB is thus a clear exception to the rule stated by Durk Pearson and Sandy Shaw in *Life Extension* that "Most drugs that increase GH [growth hormone] decrease prolactin and vice versa." In fact, as also noted in *Life Extension*, the effects of these two hormones are often diametrically opposed [Pearson & Shaw, 1982]. For instance, growth hormone is an immune stimulant, whereas excessive levels of prolactin have been attributed with anti-immune effects; where growth hormone is associated with fat reduction, prolactin is associated with fat increase; and where growth hormone is thought to have prosexual effects, the sex-negative consequences of high prolactin concentrations have been well documented.

However, it is probably safe to assume that, in the case of GHB, the effects of growth hormone release overwhelm those of prolactin release in those areas where the actions of the two hormones are opposed. While an intravenous dose of 2.5 grams of GHB can increase prolactin levels by as much as a factor of five, the same dose induces a much greater surge of growth hormone—an increase by a factor of sixteen.

It has been suggested that GHB's seemingly contradictory function as a simultaneous stimulator of growth hormone and prolactin release might be resolved through a mechanism, consistent with its inhibition of dopamine release, that involves the serotonin system. As of this time, however, such notions—extrapolated from observations involving the nervous system of a certain species of mussel—are entirely speculative [Takahara, 1977].

## Other physiological effects

In addition to its effects on concentrations of dopamine, growth hormone, and prolactin, several other aspects of GHB's physiological action are worthy of note. GHB induces what has been called "remarkable hypotonia," or muscle relaxation [Fowkes, 1993; Vickers, 1969]. GHB is completely metabolized into carbon dioxide—the primary constituent of normal human exhalation—and water, leaving the body with absolutely no residue of toxic metabolites [Vickers, 1969; Laborit, 1972]. Because of the efficiency with which it is metabolized, GHB can no longer be detected in urine four to five hours after it is taken by injection [Laborit, 1964].

GHB activates a metabolic process known as the "pentose pathway" which plays an important role in the synthesis of protein within the body [Laborit, 1972], including muscle tissue. It also features what has been called a "protein sparing" effect [Laborit, 1964], meaning that it reduces the rate at which the body breaks down its own proteins (for example, those in muscle). These properties, along with GHB's role as a growth hormone releasing agent, underlie its use as an aid to muscle building and fat loss.

Anesthetic doses of GHB are accompanied by a small increase in blood sugar levels, and a significant decrease in cholesterol. Respiration becomes slower and deeper. Blood pressure may rise or fall slightly, or remain stable, but a moderate bradycardia (slowing of the heart) is common [Vickers, 1969; Laborit, 1964]. A slight drop in body temperature also occurs [Laborit, 1964]. While these effects have been observed at anesthetic levels, it is probably safe to assume at least some similar activity takes place in response to smaller doses, if to a lesser degree. Indeed, a ten to thirteen percent decrease in heart rate has been observed among patients administered GHB in sufficiently low dosage for them to remain conscious [Gallimberti, 1989].

Most people find that 2.5 grams (one teaspoon) of GHB powder is sufficient to induce sleep.

GHB also stimulates the release of acetylcholine in the brain [Gallimberti, 1989]. This chemical is a neurotransmitter credited with an important role in memory.

## GHB, Sleep, and Narcolepsy

GHB has been called "almost an ideal sleep inducing substance" [Dean, 1993]. A sufficient dose of GHB will induce sudden sleep within five to ten minutes [Laborit, 1964].

Many other hypnotics interfere with various stages of the sleep cycle—thus preventing the body from achieving a complete and balanced session of rest and recuperation. The most remarkable facet of GHB-induced sleep is its physiological resemblance to normal sleep [Fowkes, 1993]. For instance, GHB sleep is characterized by increased levels of carbon dioxide in the arteries, as in normal sleep [Vickers, 1969]. During normal and GHB sleep, the central nervous system continues to be responsive to "noxious stimuli" (pain and other irritations), a factor which sets limits on GHB's uses in anesthesia [Vickers, 1969]. GHB facilitates both REM (rapid eye movement) sleep, considered "the most restful sleep" [Dean, 1993], and "slow-wave" (non-REM) sleep, the stage of sleep featuring increased release of growth hormone [Laborit, 1972]. And, unlike the unconsciousness induced by other anesthetics, that triggered by GHB does not feature a decrease in consumption of oxygen [Laborit, 1964].

No doubt due in large part to its resemblance to natural sleep, GHB-induced sleep lacks the morning-after "hangover" and grogginess often associated with other sleep-inducing agents. To the contrary, people usually experience a rapid—even sudden—and complete awakening from GHB sleep that leaves them feeling unusually refreshed and invigorated [Fowkes, 1993].

The primary difference between normal and GHB sleep is the length of the sleeping phase. GHB sleep tends to be more brief— from two to six hours—than what most people consider a normal night's sleep. Thus many people who use GHB for sleep awaken in the middle of the night in an alert state. Some have called this pattern the "dawn effect" and have speculated that it is related to the release of the dopamine build-up that is stored during the GHB sleep cycle.

Some who experience the "dawn effect" have found that they can avoid it by decreasing their initial bedtime dose. Others merely take a second dose when they awaken in the middle of the night, which puts them back to sleep. Some of those for whom the GHB-initiated sleep cycle is five or six hours long find themselves more than adequately refreshed by GHB sleep of such duration. They may therefore choose to take advantage of this "built-in alarm clock" by using GHB to shorten the total amount of sleep they need.

Because GHB sleep is deep and continuous, this compound is especially valuable for light sleepers troubled by frequent night-time awakenings. Such arousals have been shown to to cause fatigue and interfere with functioning during the day [Fowkes, 1993].

It should be noted that not everyone can be put to sleep by GHB. The authors have spoken to three men who have never achieved sleep even with the doses normally used for such purposes. In addition, Takahara [1977] reported that one of the six men in the growth hormone study cited above remained conscious even though he had received two and a half grams of GHB *intravenously*, a dosage which rendered the rest of the participants unconscious.

Outside of the United States, GHB's ability to induce deep and restful sleep has afforded this compound a role in the treatment of narcolepsy. Narcoleptics are sometimes given stimulants during the day to prevent spontaneous episodes of sleep. GHB treatment for narcolepsy approaches the problem from the opposite perspective. When taken orally at bedtime, GHB provides narcoleptics with deeper sleep and greater frequency of REM cycles, leading to fewer daytime narcoleptic episodes [Fadda, 1989; Chin, 1992]. Some of the "auxiliary" symptoms of narcolepsy—which GHB is also of assistance in treating—are associated with dopamine deficiency. It's possible that the daytime release of the dopamine buildup caused by use of GHB at night is the mechanism by which these symptoms are alleviated [Chin, 1992].

## GHB as a Smart Drug?

It seems unlikely that the GHB "high"—at least at greater levels of intensity—would be conducive to disciplined cognitive activity. Rather, the question regarding GHB's potential as a "smart drug" is whether or not its use for recreational, sleep-inducing, or growth hormone-related purposes in the evening or at night might facilitate cognitive and learning processes during the next day.

REM sleep and protein synthesis—processes which may be linked, and which are both facilitated by GHB—have been correlated

"GHB is the most effective, non-toxic...non-habituating, and lowest-cost sleep-inducing substance ever discovered by man."

So said Lance Griffin, a health-food-store owner sent to Federal prison for selling GHB. The quote comes from an interview performed by KTLA Los Angeles for a television news story about GHB.

KTLA also interviewed one of Griffin's customers, a woman with a severe sleep disorder to whom he had recommended and sold GHB.

"I've tried everything over-the-counter you can get," she said, "as well as I've had prescriptions for sleep medication that have been prescribed by the medical profession, and they all have adverse side effects. Using GHB permitted me to function normally again because I was able to get more than just a couple hours' sleep a night, and without any of the chemicals and side effects that the over-the-counter and prescribed medications used to give me. Lance was a guardian angel in disguise...I had no idea that anything existed like GHB on the planet. And I was in Heaven when I found out about it." Now deprived of GHB because of the FDA ban, she proclaimed, *"I'd do anything to get back in touch with GHB."*

with periods of intensive learning [Laborit, 1972]. As mentioned earlier, GHB has also been shown to stimulate the release of acetylcholine, one of the brain's own "smart chemicals" [Gallimberti, 1989]. These effects suggest a possible role for GHB as a cognition-enhancer.

Beyond possible specific mechanisms is a more general route by which GHB might improve cognitive function. A good night's sleep improves cognitive ability while sleep deprivation impairs it. Since GHB facilitates and deepens sleep, it seems likely that it would also promote mental acuity.

The authors have encountered only one study directly relevant to GHB and cognition. Here, subjects *under the influence of GHB* scored "no worse" than controls on a word fluency test. (At least GHB didn't make them *dumber.*) This result is particularly interesting since most sedative drugs impair cognition.

## GHB, Fat Reduction and Muscle Building

Both activation of the pentose pathway and release of growth hormone offer means by which GHB could be expected to increase the ratio of lean tissue to fat. While there is a great deal of anecdotal evidence that GHB can be used effectively both for weight loss and muscle building, on-line database searches performed for this book produced no documentation of scientific studies on GHB and weight loss.

According to articles in body-building magazines, athletes have experienced increases in strength and decreases in fat as a result of GHB. And one man in his thirties interviewed for this book shared his enthusiasm for the results of his girlfriend's use of GHB for muscle-building and fat-loss purposes:

> "*It's made a huge difference in her breasts. They're higher, and it's made her pectoral muscles hard and firm. And it's given her great back muscles. All of this even though she doesn't really work out that much.*"

Such reports are not unusual among those using GHB for its growth hormone effects.

## GHB and Exercise-Related Stress

Animal experiments provide support for anecdotal evidence suggesting that GHB can be used to increase muscular strength as well as endurance and the overall capacity for hard physical work. In studies with rats, GHB ameliorated stress to the body and muscles incurred as a result of physical labor, positively affecting biochemistry, muscle structure, and metabolism. Among GHB's benefits in this regard is a decrease in the amount of lactic acid, responsible for the muscular soreness (or "burn") generated by exercise. As a result of such effects, in one study the rats' capacity for physical work progressively increased across the fifteen to sixty day time periods during which GHB was administered [Kleimenova, 1979; Ostravskaya, 1982].

## GHB, Alcohol and Alcoholism

GHB shows great promise in the treatment of alcoholism. In Europe, one of its primary uses is to relieve withdrawal symptoms, cravings, and anxiety among alcoholics.

Physical alcohol dependence can be generated in rats by administering alcohol according to a program that consistently maintains high blood levels for a period of several days. When their alcohol input is discontinued, rats subjected to such a regimen develop, within a few hours, a withdrawal syndrome closely

GHB could play a role not only in the treatment of alcoholism but in its prevention among those who might be vulnerable to it. This possibility is suggested by a study of rats in whom a strong preference for alcohol (a sort of "pre-alcoholic" condition) had been established. These rats consistently reduced their consumption of alcohol when GHB was made available as an alternative [Gallimberti, 1989.]

resembling that exhibited by humans, including tremors, convulsions, and hypersensitivity to sound [Fadda, 1989].

In 1989, such rats were used in an investigation of GHB's ability to treat the symptoms of alcohol withdrawal. In this test, a sufficiently high dose of GHB succeeded in suppressing *all withdrawal symptoms* [Fadda, 1989].

In the same year, a similar study was conducted with human alcoholics according to a methodologically rigorous, double-blind, placebo-controlled format. The treatment was enormously successful. After the first administration of GHB, "nearly all withdrawal symptoms disappeared within two to seven hours..." The subjects in this study were given steadily decreasing doses of GHB for seven days. During this entire period, the intensity of withdrawal syndrome, measured on a scale of 0 to 3, remained below 2, the rating designated for "moderate."

Several of GHB's properties suggest an enormous, and largely overlooked, usefulness in psychotherapeutic and psychiatric arenas.

The only side effect observed was slight, occasional, and transient dizziness. The researchers concluded, "the results clearly indicated that GHB is effective for the suppression of withdrawal symptoms in alcoholics" [Gallimberti, 1989].

Administration of GHB has been found to prevent alcohol consumption among rats that otherwise tend to ingest alcohol voluntarily [Fadda, 1989; Gallimberti, 1989]. In light of this finding and the results of the other alcohol-related studies recounted here, it seems likely that GHB could function similarly among humans, serving as an effective, non-toxic substitute for those with a strong attraction to alcohol (as it did in the "angel" anecdote in the gray box near the beginning of this chapter).

Nonetheless, in the United States, over-the-counter sale of GHB—a substance of remarkably low toxicity that has been clearly demonstrated to exert a diversity of health-enhancing effects—continues to be prohibited. Meanwhile, a smorgasbord of products containing alcohol—a highly toxic compound whose degenerative and often fatal physiological and psychological effects are well-known—continues to be readily available at every corner liquor store. How can such a situation be explained, let alone justified?

## Other Uses of GHB

GHB is clearly a compound of enormous versatility for both clinical and "alternative" uses. Even the rather extensive discussion provided so far has not yet exhausted the variety of ways in which GHB has been or might be employed. This section will briefly summarize those applications not yet covered.

### *Anesthesia*

GHB has been used for decades as a general anesthetic. Administered intravenously, an anesthetic dose of GHB is in the range of 60 to 70 milligrams per kilogram of body weight (for a 150-pound person this would be 4.1-4.8 grams) [Vickers, 1969]. Its advantages as an anesthetic include low toxicity, relatively few contraindications, slowing of the heart rate without loss of blood pressure, the absence of irritation to the veins with intravenous administration, muscle relaxation, usual absence of respiratory depression, and reduction of body temperature or "hypothermia." By reducing the metabolic demands of the brain, hypothermia offers a "protective" effect regarding certain possible complications during surgery. GHB also performs various other protective and anti-shock functions of value in surgical situations [Laborit, 1964; Vickers, 1969].

However, GHB can almost never be used in anesthesia without the additional administration of other drugs [Vickers, 1969] because it does not produce complete surgical anesthesia except in children [Laborit, 1964]. The autonomic nervous system remains active during GHB-induced anesthesia, and thus the body continues to respond to surgical stimuli through increases in heart rate, blood pressure, and cardiac output, as well as through sweating, peripheral vasoconstriction, vocalization, and reflex muscle action [Vickers, 1969]. Local anesthetics or other drugs which suppress these responses must therefore also be used, but concomitant use of GHB can allow for much smaller doses of these depressants [Vickers, 1969]. The use of GHB in combination with a local anesthetic is comparable to the way a dentist or orthodontic surgeon might use Novocaine to kill pain in the mouth along with nitrous oxide to render the patient unconscious during the procedure.

## Obstetrics

GHB has gained some popularity as an obstetric anesthetic in Italy and France [Vickers, 1969]. It has been attributed with "spectacular action on the dilation of the cervix" [Laborit, 1964]. Other attributes of GHB that can be valuable in childbirth include decreased anxiety, greater intensity and frequency of uterine contractions, increased sensitivity to oxytocic drugs (used to induce contractions), preservation of reflexes, a lack of respiratory depression in the fetus, and protection against cardiac anoxia (which could be especially important when the fetus' oxygen supply is threatened by "wrapping" of the umbilical cord around the neck) [Vickers, 1969; Laborit, 1964].

## Psychiatry and psychotherapy

Positive results concerning GHB's efficacy in treating anxiety have been demonstrated in tests involving schizophrenic subjects [Laborit, 1964], and its sedative properties have earned it a role as a psychotherapeutic adjunct [Vickers, 1969]. It has also been used to assist the process of "abreaction," or the release (usually through verbalization) of repressed emotion [Vickers, 1969].

GHB has a strong "anxiolytic" (or anti-anxiety) effect and is far less toxic and addictive than most substances commonly used for this purpose. Furthermore, the reduction of inhibitions, tendency to verbalize, and lack of fear characteristic of the GHB "high" would seem to provide an ideal context for the verbal exploration of difficult emotional territory during therapy—a process often hampered by fear, inhibition, or general shyness. (Not surprisingly, there are many anecdotal reports of psychological breakthroughs associated with GHB, particularly during the early period of use.)

GHB may also prove to have value in couples therapy. This compound would seem promising as a facilitator among partners of intimate verbal communication when it has become "blocked" in important areas, much as MDMA was once used by many couples' counselors before it was banned. It could also be used as an aide to overcoming sexual and sensual barriers that may be interfering with the relationship. (The story of the "GHB angel" in the gray box towards the beginning of this chapter serves as an example of both of these potential uses.)

### Life extension

The eminent gerontologist Ward Dean, MD has speculated that GHB "may even have life-extension potential" [Dean, 1993], and a prominent psychiatrist has referred to its "youth-enhancing" effects. Prior to the recent development of GHB's "recreational" and night-club market, life extension enthusiasts constituted one of the few circles in which this drug was well-known. However, the authors have found no references to scientific studies directly investigating GHB's efficacy as a life-extender *per se*.

Aside from its general anti-stress and recuperative properties, much of GHB's promise in life extension lies in its potency as a releaser of growth hormone. GHB could, perhaps, be used to combat the age-related decline in output of this hormone, which plays vital roles in immunity and many other areas. Furthermore, sleep disorders are especially prevalent among the elderly, and may well accelerate their aging process. GHB could be used to treat—and conceivably even to prevent—age-related sleep dysfunction, and in this capacity could quite possibly extend lives.

### Anti-convulsant

Despite the fact that, as noted earlier, clonic movements can sometimes be a side effect of GHB, this compound can also function as an anti-convulsant. Sufficient doses have been shown to protect rats against convulsions produced both by pressurized oxygen and by a number of convulsion-inducing drugs [Laborit, 1964].

### Cerebral and vascular "protective" effects

GHB may protect the brain and heart during conditions which depress vital functions or decrease oxygen availability. In animal studies, GHB has extended survival time under conditions of low oxygen supply (or "hypoxia") up to eighty-five percent [Artru, 1980], and has increased the survival time of the mouse heart when completely deprived of oxygen ("anoxia") [Vickers, 1969]. (However, unlike all other known anesthetics, GHB does *not* result in an overall decrease in oxygen consumption by the body [Laborit, 1964].) GHB also protects against various kinds of arrhythmia (irregularity of heartbeat) that can be induced in animals [Vickers, 1969; Laborit, 1964].

It is suspected that part of GHB's cerebral protective function involves slowing down the metabolism of brain cells and thus reducing their requirements for oxygen and glucose [Chin, 1992; Artru, 1980]. These effects are part of a hibernation-like anesthetic condition assisted by GHB's capacity to induce mild "hypothermia," or reduction in body temperature. Another factor in GHB's anti-shock capability may be the marked vasodilation induced in the liver and kidney areas, thus increasing blood flow to those vital regions.

One man in his early thirties who has used GHB extensively for sexual purposes says, "it makes sex feel truly intense, especially when you first start using it, and I suspect it makes sex feel better for a day or two after."

Another remarkable "protective" property of GHB is that it increases the survival rates of animals exposed to radiation [Laborit, 1964].

## GHB and Sex

Among the wide variety of substances used by the many people who were interviewed for this book, no other compound consistently generated a level of enthusiasm regarding prosexual properties comparable to that surrounding GHB.

As discussed elsewhere in this book, the scientific and medical communities have traditionally been extremely reluctant to ascribe aphrodisiac properties to any substance, although this tendency may have abated somewhat in recent years. It is a testament, then, to the power of GHB's sexual effects that they were clearly acknowledged—if only in hesitating phrases and elliptical language—in the scientific literature as early as 1972.

In a paper published in January of that year, Dr. Laborit, the French researcher who first synthesized GHB, wrote:

> *"A last point should still be mentioned: the [GHB] action on man which could be called 'aphrodisiac.' We cannot present any animal experiments on this subject. However, the oral form has now been sufficiently used so that, as generally agreed, no doubt can subsist as to its existence."*

After this provocative statement, Laborit offers no elaboration aside from brief speculation as to the nature of the underlying biological mechanism of GHB's sexual effects (a subject taken up at the end of this section).

Four central prosexual properties clearly emerge from an overview of the anecdotal data gathered from interviews and other sources. These are disinhibition, heightening of the sense of touch, enhancement of male erectile capacity, and increased power of orgasm.

### Disinhibition

Perhaps the foremost prosexual property of GHB is disinhibition. Some users suggest that GHB's other sexual benefits are secondary effects made possible by this loosening and relaxation of psychosomatic constraint.

A number of people have commented that disinhibition from GHB is particularly marked among women. A man who has used GHB with a variety of female partners describes this compound as "a profound disinhibitor for women." His observation is echoed by a female researcher who has collected a great deal of technical as well as anecdotal and experiential data on GHB: "A lot of women say it helps their libido because of the disinhibition."

A woman in her early thirties had been using GHB as an aid to sleep. When she heard about its disinhibiting effects on sexuality, she thought that it might help her and her new partner overcome the "tentative and nervous quality that comes from being with somebody new." She reports:

> "*Inhibitions were definitely gone. It made me more aggressive, and definitely helped us break through some barriers. After the GHB started to kick in, it was just really easy to go for it.*"

One male who has experimented extensively with GHB in group sex contexts describes the results as "wonderfully loose."

### Tactility

As a male user put it, "the sense of touch becomes electric or sparkling" with GHB. One woman—who described a scene in which her and her partner spent a long stretch of time exploring the pleasures of touching a sheepskin rug—attributes GHB with "enhanced sensuality and intense eroticism. You can get lost in what something feels like—not only how things feel to the touch, but how your whole body feels when it's being touched."

### Erection

Many men report that GHB helps them to achieve erection more quickly, and makes their erections firmer, more stable, and longer-lasting. As one man put it, "GHB really helps to sustain erection. Something that would normally distract you just doesn't."

In her book *Love Potions*, Cynthia Mervis Watson, MD relates an anecdote involving a man in his seventies who "took GHB and noticed a return of his morning erections, which had disappeared for many years following cardiac surgery" [Watson, 1993]. A male scholar in his fifties, who sometimes has spontaneous erections on GHB even in the absence of sexual stimulation, compares and contrasts the effects of this drug with those of MDMA (or "Ecstasy"): "With GHB, I get both warm and cuddly, like you do with Ecstasy, and hard and crusty, like you don't."

### Orgasm and ejaculation

Women often report that GHB makes their orgasms longer and more intense—as well as more difficult or time-consuming to achieve, especially at higher doses. One forty-one year old songwriter and single mother who has sometimes "had a hard time coming on GHB" tells of one occasion when she "took a very small quantity—an eighth of a teaspoon. Although I didn't get 'high' and couldn't really feel *anything* from the drug, I had this incredibly long orgasm that was quite unusual."

As with its other effects, GHB's impact on female orgasm seems highly sensitive to small adjustments in dosage. A biochemist who has collected data on GHB says, "higher doses can postpone orgasm. I've heard complaints from women that if the amount isn't *just right*, or if they've had too much, they have trouble with orgasm. The effect is very dose-dependent."

GHB's effects on male ejaculation also seem to bear a close relationship to dosage. One man reports, "It can become very hard to come if you take a tiny bit too much." When GHB was still sold over-the-counter, one company advertised its GHB product with the claim that it "markedly delays ejaculation." Apparently, at slightly higher dosage levels, this *delay* can be experienced as *interference*.

This occasional interference with orgasm, however, does *not* seem to interfere to any great extent with users' enjoyment of sex under the influence of GHB. Most feel that a GHB-charged orgasm is well worth the extra wait and work that it may entail. The young woman whose experiments with GHB and sexual disinhibition were described above said, "I did find it harder to come, it took a little longer. But it seems to really enhance orgasm... everything's just going on up in your head...it's hard to explain!"

### Other sex-related effects

It has been mentioned elsewhere that the disinhibition associated with GHB can lead to an increase in undefended verbal disclosure. Couples and sex partners using GHB may find it easier to discuss tender, sensitive, and previously guarded emotional issues—an effect that has been compared to that of MDMA. This enhancement of verbal communication can lead to stronger feelings of emotional intensity, intimacy, and bondedness or "heart-connection" during sex.

It is also worth noting that GHB has sometimes been attributed with the capacity to increase clitoral and vaginal sensitivity.

### Possible mechanisms for GHB's prosexual properties

What biochemical mechanism might underlie GHB's aphrodisiac effects?

The disinhibition which seems to occur as part of GHB's "hypnotic" effect is probably one of the most important factors leading to GHB's aphrodisiac action. But endocrine and other factors may be significant as well.

Drugs that increase dopamine levels often have sex-enhancing effects. However, as mentioned earlier, greater dopamine *activity* is not associated with GHB's augmentation of cerebral dopamine concentrations. It is therefore unlikely that this compound's effects on dopamine can be held directly responsible for its prosexual action.

However, it has been speculated that GHB's dopamine-related effects might lead to a decrease in serotonin levels. The latter neurotransmitter is often attributed with anti-sexual properties, partly due to observations that serotonin-depleting compounds such as pCPA facilitate sexual activity in animals. Such possible anti-serotonin action might account for some of GHB's prosexual properties [Laborit, 1972].

In contrast to conjectured effects on the serotonin system, GHB's potent stimulation of growth hormone release is well-documented [Takahara, 1977; Fowkes, 1993]. Strong anecdotal evidence points towards aphrodisiac effects on the part of growth hormone and growth hormone releasers. Thus GHB's growth hormone-related effects provide an additional possible explanation for its prosexual qualities.

As mentioned earlier, levels of the neurotransmitter acetylcholine rise in response to GHB. This effect may well serve as one of the mechanisms underlying GHB's ability to promote firm and long-lasting erections, as acetylcholine is thought to play a significant role in erectile physiology [PDR, 1994].

GHB is also a vasodilator, an agent which expands blood vessels and therefore increases blood supply to those areas of the body in which vasodilation occurs. As mentioned earlier, strong vasodilatory action of GHB has been observed in the regions of the liver and kidney [Laborit, 1964]. If this effect extends to the nearby genital area, it could further account for GHB's prosexual properties, particularly with regard to male erection and female genital sensitivity.

At the same time that GHB prevents the *release* of dopamine *from* brain cells, it *increases* the rate at which this neurotransmitter is manufactured *within* brain cells [Cash, 1994; Cooper 1974]. Between this increased synthesis of dopamine during the period of GHB's activity, and the large release of stored dopamine suspected to occur as GHB wears off, it seems almost certain that dopamine activity is greater *after* a GHB session than it was *before*. Thus, in spite of the short-term dopamine-dampening property of this compound, GHB probably has the *net effect* of a dopamine-boosting agent. Such an increase in subsequent dopamine activity might be responsible for a more long-range prosexual effect in addition to the short-term sex-enhancement discussed in most of the anecdotes in this chapter.

It is indeed peculiar that a substance known to stimulate short-term surges of prolactin (a hormone implicated in decreased libido, impotence, and other sexual problems), and which probably actually *decreases* dopamine activity, should demonstrate such marked aphrodisiac qualities. It seems likely that the combination of disinhibition and growth hormone release—perhaps along with vasodilation and possible anti-serotonin action—simply overwhelms those actions of GHB that would tend to predict anti-sexual results. It's also entirely possible that the primary mechanism of GHB's prosexual effects has not yet been identified.

In any case, at least one aspect of GHB's aphrodisiac properties is not in doubt: for most people *it works*.

## Legal Status and Availability

*Note:* _____

As we are going to press with this book, the legal status and availability of GHB is in flux. The FDA says it is banned, yet one US pharmacy (legally, they say) is making it available by prescription. By the time you read this the situation may have changed. Our suggestion is that you send us the tearout card at the front of this book and request our *Directory of Mail Order Pharmacies* and *Directory of Physicians*. These listings are kept up to date and, if there are any legal sources for GHB, you will find them there.

At the time of this writing, GHB has been banned from over-the-counter sale in the US. However, it has not been legally scheduled like those controlled substances falling within the purview of the DEA. These conditions leave GHB in a legal twilight zone in the United States. While there is technically no illegality attached to the possession or sale of GHB—and it continues to be available to legitimate laboratories and scientists for research purposes—selling it specifically for human consumption, especially while making claims about its health benefits, can constitute a violation of FDA strictures. (Simple personal possession and use, on the other hand, should at least theoretically incur no legal risk.)

The status of GHB in the US is comparable to that of the amino acid tryptophan. Until a few years ago, tryptophan was widely available in health food stores, pharmacies, and even grocery stores. After its use was linked to incidents of an unusual blood disorder, over-the-counter sales of tryptophan were restricted and subsequently banned by the FDA. Although these cases were definitively traced to impurities present in only a few batches produced by a single company using an unconventional manufacturing process, the ban was never lifted. To this day, tryptophan is still unavailable—even by prescription—in the United States.

Despite the fact that GHB is not technically a controlled substance, those involved in the manufacture, distribution and sale of GHB should be forewarned. One chemist who attempted to comply with FDA guidelines while making and selling GHB has nonetheless been prosecuted and imprisoned. He cautions: "The FDA has been programmatically harassing people involved in the sale of GHB and busting them on any charge they can get away with."

The situation regarding GHB and the law is yet fluid. While possession is still legal at the time of this writing, the intense controversy surrounding GHB could easily fuel Federal scheduling in the near future. Meanwhile, individual states may independently pass their own statutes against GHB.

The peculiar legal status of GHB in the United States leaves those who wish to acquire it for personal consumption with little means to do so except by way of personal connection to the informal, semi-underground network. Presently, GHB seems to be widely available—and growing in popularity—via this "gray market." Since most of the GHB available through such channels is of the "bootleg" variety, manufactured by non-professional "kitchen" chemists, concerns about quality and purity become paramount. *Caveat emptor* (buyer beware!).

*(Note: In various European and other nations, GHB is available by prescription. Doctors, pharmacists, or government agencies in locations where GHB has been granted a legal status different from that in U.S. should be able to provide specific information on GHB's legality and availability in their respective countries.)*

## Determining Purity and Quality

A chemist who has examined various batches of bootleg GHB warns that "there is a lot of bad stuff out there." He has found everything from "dog hair to sodium hydroxide" in GHB products, and has noted that some "street" GHB is manufactured using recycled industrial ingredients, a process which can result in the presence of toxic heavy metals in the product. (The research for this book, however, has produced no clear cases of adverse effects attributable to impurities in "street" GHB),

This chemist recommends purchasing GHB only in pow-dered—as opposed to liquid—form. "If someone is sophisticated enough to produce the granular product," he advises, "they probably know what they're doing."

Pure GHB powder can be recognized by a number of characteristics. It has a salty/licorice flavor, and is at first chalky in texture but becomes greasy when rubbed between the fingers. It is very "hygroscopic," meaning that it readily absorbs water. Thus, when a small quantity is left out in open air overnight, it will turn into a puddle (unless you live in a desert-dry area.) Pure GHB powder will completely dissolve in a sufficient quantity of water; any particles that do not dissolve represent some kind of impurity.

Keep in mind that the purity of "street" or gray market GHB is not an issue which played a role in *prompting* the FDA ban, but rather is a *consequence* of it. Such matters would be of considerably less concern if GHB were still available over-the-counter from manufacturers practicing quality control and using a brand name whose reputation they desired to uphold.

As of 1994, 100 gram bottles of GHB sold in the range of fifty to eighty dollars.

## Safety Issues

As has been emphasized, the overall safety of GHB is well-established, and no deaths attributable to GHB have been reported over the thirty year period that this compound has been in use [Vickers, 1969; Chin, 1992]. In fact, as of 1990, only forty-six adverse reactions had been reported in the United States—surely constituting only an infinitesimal fraction of actual usage—all followed by rapid and complete recovery [Chin, 1992]. Unlike a large proportion of other drugs—including alcohol and even Tylenol—GHB has no toxic effects on the liver, kidney, or other organs [Vickers, 1969; Chin, 1992].

A number of long-term human studies not yet discussed seem

to leave the basic safety of this compound beyond doubt. One program of sleep therapy using six to eight grams daily for a period of eight to ten days produced *no* side effects. One researcher even reports that doses as high as twenty to thirty grams per twenty-four hour period have been used for several days without negative consequences [Vickers, 1969] (although such a level for self-experimentation is certainly *not* recommended). In the Canadian studies of narcolepsy mentioned earlier, the nightly use of two to six teaspoons (one teaspoon equalling roughly 2.5 grams) for several years resulted in neither in reports of long-term adverse effects nor problems with issues of addiction or dependence when use of the substance was discontinued. (See "Addictive potential" at the end of this section.) In one of these studies, a patient inadvertently ingested *fifteen teaspoons* without adverse consequence "other than deep sedation and headache the next day" [Chin, 1992]. And in France, sub-anesthetic oral doses were used by "a large number of patients for about six years" without untoward effect [Laborit, 1972].

The "LD 50" ("lethal dose 50%," or the dosage level fatal to half of those to whom it is administered) for GHB in rats has been calculated at 1.70 grams per kilogram of body weight [Laborit, 1964], which is in the range of five to fifteen times the anesthetic dose [Vickers, 1969]. Some have even questioned whether the animal deaths that occur at these dosage levels are due to the active drug itself or to sodium poisoning from the salt form in which it is administered [Vickers, 1969]. As one researcher has pointed out, if sodium toxicity is indeed the cause of rat fatality, it becomes safe to say that GHB is "less toxic than table salt." Rats injected daily for seventy days with one-tenth of the LD 50 have shown no significant differences from a control group [Laborit, 1964].

Extrapolating from the data on rats, the human LD 50 would be around 115 grams for a 150 lb person—a quantity about fifty times that usually required to induce sleep in most people. Although such extrapolations are frequently unreliable due to differences in absorption between rats and human beings, this information nonetheless points towards a remarkable safety profile for GHB.

### No driving, no chainsaws

GHB is classified as a sedative-hypnotic. Its effects will therefore bear some similarity to those of other hypnotics like tranquilizers and alcohol. GHB not only "*may* cause drowsiness" like these other drugs—it will *almost inevitably* do so. Ataxia, or discoordination, can also be a side effect of GHB. Therefore, the following warning is in order:

*Do not drive or operate dangerous machinery while under the influence of GHB.*

### Side effects

One researcher has characterized the action of GHB as "without serious side effects," and some research programs have reported *no side effects at all*. Nonetheless, it's clear that side effects can occur. Those most commonly experienced are drowsiness, dizziness, nausea, and sometimes vomiting. Headache is sometimes reported. As mentioned, clonic movements (muscle spasms or "seizures") have been observed during the onset of GHB-induced sleep. Some ataxia (or discoordination) is not uncommon. As discussed in the section on "The Action of GHB in the Body," a moderate slowing of the heart-rate is a common, and small changes in blood pressure can take place. At very high doses, cardiac and respiratory depression can occur. Orthostatic hypotension (a sudden drop in blood pressure upon standing up quickly, recognizable by a brief dizziness) has also been reported.

More unusual and extreme reactions have included diarrhea, lack of bladder control, temporary amnesia, and sleepwalking. More side effects can occur when GHB is combined with central nervous system depressants [Chin, 1992, Gallimberti, 1989; Takahara, 1977; Vickers, 1969].

Anecdotal evidence suggests that most "recreational" users of GHB do not usually experience unpleasant side effects. Furthermore, it should be emphasized that such effects can generally be avoided by careful and informed self-administration (see below).

### Contraindications

Contraindications for GHB have been described as "remarkably few" [Vickers, 1969]. Those who suffer from any of the following conditions should not use GHB: severe illness of any kind; epilepsy; eclampsia (convulsions); bradycardia (slowed heart-beat) due to conduction problems (left-bundle-branch-block is an example of conduction difficulty); Cushing's syndrome; severe cardiovascular disease; and severe hypertension [Dean, 1993; Gallimberti, 1989; Vickers, 1969].

Severe alcoholism is sometimes mentioned as a contraindication for GHB [Dean, 1993], even though GHB has been used quite successfully in the treatment of withdrawal among alcoholics. The explanation for this seeming contradiction probably lies in the assumption that severe alcoholics are likely to ignore precautions against combining GHB with alcohol.

Because GHB stimulates a short-term surge of prolactin, those suffering from hyperprolactinemia may have reason to avoid GHB. (Please see the chapter on bromocriptine.)

### Combinations

Most of the extreme cases of adverse reaction recounted in the section entitled "Setting the Record Straight" involved the use of central nervous system depressants in addition to GHB. The effects of GHB are strongly potentiated by such compounds (and *vice versa*). CNS depressants include benzodiazepines ("minor tranquilizers" such as Valium and Xanax), phenothiazines ("major tranquilizers" like Thorazine and Stellazine), various painkillers (opiates like codeine and barbiturates like phenobarbital), alcohol, and even many over-the-counter allergy and sleep remedies. Mixing GHB with such medications seems to increase the likelihood of adverse reactions [Chin, 1992; Laborit, 1964.] A simple, straightforward caution is in order:

*Don't mix GHB with depressants.*

### Sudden unconsciousness

As one experienced user of GHB warns, "it can make you fall asleep at inappropriate times and places." This is the most potentially problematic aspect of GHB use. The amount that will leave a given individual suddenly and totally unconscious within fifteen minutes or less is usually less than twice the amount required to give the same person a pleasant, manageable prosexual "high." This rather steep "dose-response curve" results in a narrow threshold that can be inadvertently crossed rather easily, particularly for the inexperienced user.

A number of anecdotes illustrate the potential conse-quences—from humorous to alarming—that mismanagement of GHB's "unconsciousness threshold" can create.

One man lay down on his bed while brushing his teeth after taking GHB—and awoke some hours later, the toothbrush still in his mouth.

Another man tells of an incident during a GHB-enhanced group-sex episode: "We were all gathered around one woman who was lying on the rug, touching her, the entire group giving her all our attention. She kept saying, 'Oh, this feels so good, I can't believe how good it feels.' Another woman in the group fell asleep right on top of her. So we carefully lifted her up and put her in the bed."

Complications can arise when a person who has accidentally fallen into the deepest stage of GHB sleep is encountered by others who become unduly alarmed because they don't know the reason why he or she can't be aroused. In one instance, a man who had taken a few swigs of liquid GHB couldn't make it to his bedroom, and crumpled to unconsciousness at the bottom of the stairs. When his housemates—who had no idea he'd taken GHB—discovered him in this condition, they were understandably concerned, called 911, and had him taken to the emergency room. Predictably enough, he awoke suddenly in fine condition shortly after arrival at the hospital, wondering what all the fuss was about.

In talking to users of GHB, the authors have encountered a number of tales of this kind. One experienced experimenter, a woman in her early thirties who uses GHB for enhancement of both sleep and sex, offers the following succinct statement of a constructive attitude towards this drug: "It's not a toy. It's not going to kill you, but it can knock you out for a while. You have to be safe and conscientious."

### Addictive potential

Although studies have strongly suggested that addictive properties are absent with GHB, a warning is nevertheless in order. If enough people use almost any substance, there will be those who develop an addictive, unhealthy, or otherwise counterproductive relationship with it. GHB is no exception.

We have heard several stories of people using GHB in a very regular—perhaps habitual—way. But, until very recently, all these people reported their habits to be quite benign: never did their GHB use visibly interfere in their lives and, when they ran out of GHB, they experienced no withdrawal symptoms.

Recently, however, we heard of one woman who clearly developed an abusive relationship with this compound. She used GHB on a continuous basis throughout the day, every day. She began to lie, when necessary, to get it. And she found herself unable to quit when she decided to do so. Over the next few years we will probably hear more such stories.

## Administration

This section consists largely of a summation of the "folk wisdom" or "street lore" that has come to surround the use of GHB. These guidelines, the cumulative result of hundreds, perhaps thousands, of personal experiments on the part of a large number of people, are well worth heeding. They offer the novice user of GHB the opportunity to bypass much of the "error" usually involved in "trial and error."

### Using a safe place

Especially during early experimentation with GHB, it is essential to use a safe location—primarily one in which sudden, unexpected unconsciousness, should it occur, will not pose a serious problem. Public situations, such as parties or nightclubs, are obviously inappropriate.

The best place is probably the bedroom of your own home (or that of a good friend or partner), or any other room containing a large, comfortable bed or sofa. After each dose of GHB, position yourself comfortably on the bed or couch and wait at least twenty minutes before getting up and moving around. If the dose is going to result in sudden unconsciousness, it will do so within this time period. Being on the bed or couch will ensure comfort and prevent injury from falling, stumbling, or dropping to the ground.

If at all appropriate, let the people around you know that you are experimenting with GHB. Tell them that they might find you in a state of sleep from which you can't be awakened, and that if this happens, your condition will pass in a few hours. Such communication may prevent unnecessary panic on their part.

### Dosage

Determining one's own appropriate dosage level is probably the trickiest aspect of working with GHB. The amount required for a given level of effect will vary from person to person. The slightest overestimation can have consequences ranging in seriousness from ruining your plans for the evening to waking up in the emergency ward as a result of panic on the part of concerned but uninformed friends or relatives.

Once you have found the levels that give you the effects you desire, they will remain consistent, as no tolerance towards GHB develops over time. However, recent alcohol consumption may decrease the effect of a given dose of GHB because these two compounds are "cross-tolerant." This means that prior ingestion of alcohol will reduce the intensity of GHB's sedative and anesthetic effects. (Here "prior ingestion" refers to alcohol consumption far back enough in time that the primary alcohol effects will have worn off. If you take GHB while still "high" from alcohol, the effects of both drugs are likely to become intensified—perhaps dangerously so.) This cross-tolerance has been demonstrated in a study with rats wherein dosages sufficient to render other rats fully unconscious caused only moderate sedation among those accustomed to a high level of alcohol intake [Fadda, 1989].

GHB should be taken on an empty stomach, preferably three to four hours after your last meal. A full stomach will delay the onset of effects, resulting in the possibility of taking an unnecessary second dose before the first dose kicks in, and may also increase the likelihood of nausea or vomiting. It is also known that prior "fasting" potentiates GHB's effects [Laborit, 1964].

Doses of GHB can be measured and controlled very accurately and conveniently by dissolving powdered GHB in purified or distilled water in a measured solution. If the number of grams of GHB is equal to the number of teaspoons of water, then, of course, a liquid will be produced one teaspoon of which will contain very close to one gram of GHB. For instance, ten grams of GHB could be dissolved in ten teaspoons of water, or 100 grams of GHB could be dissolved in 100 teaspoons. In the absence of such a solution, dosage can be determined by remembering that *one level teaspoon of GHB powder is equivalent to approximately two and a half grams*.

Here's a story that underscores the importance of taking GHB on a fairly empty stomach. One man took a full 2.5 gram dose of GHB right after eating a good portion of popcorn. After an hour he didn't feel anything, so he took another full dose. Within another hour he felt the GHB effect far more strongly than ever before.

Apparently, the popcorn soaked up the GHB like a sponge, creating a sort of time-release mechanism.

Whatever the cause, he later described the effect as "extremely unpleasant." He vomited so violently that the memory of this experience prevented him from taking GHB again for several months.

As one experienced GHB experimenter strongly recommends, "start with the smallest amount you can try; it's always best to take as little as you can." Beginning with as small a dose as possible, you can then work your way up in tiny increments, leaving plenty of time—about an hour—between administrations. One-eighth or one-quarter of a gram could serve as a starting point. This dosage could then be repeated on an hourly basis until a desirable level of "high" (or sleep, if that is the goal) has been achieved.

A first experiment performed according to these guidelines allows you to determine how favorable your individual response to the drug is, and whether or not it will tend to give you side effects. This approach will also help to minimize the intensity and duration of any negative reactions that might arise. If this first test has favorable results—or no results at all, a possibility when using such tiny quantities—you might consider doubling the size of your dosage increments for the next experiment, using a quarter or a half gram every hour.

The following point has been repeatedly emphasized by the GHB users interviewed for this report: Acquiring the experience necessary to be able to dose yourself accurately entails a period of investigation requiring patience, care, close attention, and acute self-observation.

For a third experiment, another eighth or quarter of a gram could be added to each dose. Proceeding in this fashion, slowly and carefully adding to the increments of dosage across a series of experiments, will allow you eventually to find out how much GHB you require—and can easily tolerate—in a single dose to achieve the level of effect that you find most enjoyable and useful.

Most people find that a dose in the range of three quarters to one and a half grams is suitable for prosexual purposes, and that a quantity in the range of two and a half grams is sufficient to induce sleep. Those interested in maximizing growth hormone release will derive the greatest benefit by taking a sleep-inducing dose at bedtime (for further details of practical relevance, review the section entitled "GHB, Sleep, and Narcolepsy"). Between these dosage levels is often a zone in which the GHB "high" intensifies to a point that it is no longer manageable for sexual purposes and is characterized by giddiness, decreased verbal coherence, and discoordination. Such a state is often followed shortly by sleep. Otherwise, since the GHB "high" is fairly short-lived, it is likely to settle into a more subtle level of consciousness-alteration within an hour or so.

### Countering the effects

If on any occasion you find that you are not enjoying GHB's effects, or if for any other reason you wish to discontinue or diminish the "high," there are two approaches you can use. One method is to eat; a small or medium-sized meal will usually result in rapid dissipation of effects. A strong cup of coffee or other beverage containing a significant quantity of caffeine is often all that is needed to counter the drowsiness that accompanies GHB (a mild euphoria may linger). In fact, there is scientific evidence that caffeine, a dopaminergic compound, blocks GHB's dopamine-related effects [Chin, 1992].

### The potassium question

There is some debate as to whether GHB consistently lowers potassium levels in the human body. Because of early evidence of sharp potassium loss, it was at one time considered mandatory to administer potassium supplements with GHB. Later research, however, showed only slight changes in serum potassium levels in humans, and one investigation found no differences at all. One researcher has suggested that the original evidence showing marked drops in potassium levels was influenced by the presence of other potassium-depleting drugs among a large proportion of those patients from whom the data was collected [Vickers, 1969].

To further confuse matters, animal studies have resulted in unchanged potassium levels in mice [Artru, 1980], but decreased quantities among dogs [Laborit, 1964].

While potassium supplementation is probably unnecessary for most people [Vickers, 1969], there is no harm in being on the safe side by taking a potassium supplement when you use GHB. Sources urging such a practice recommend that a quantity of potassium's elemental form should be taken that is equal to ten percent of the weight of the amount of GHB ingested. Slightly less than twenty percent of the potassium in most commercial supplements is of the elemental variety; thus, a 500 milligrams potassium tablet usually contains at most 100 milligrams of elemental potassium. Since 100 milligrams is ten percent of one gram, the formula mentioned above would require taking one such 500 milligrams potassium tablet with every gram of GHB ingested.

## Physicians and Product Sources

Please note the tearout card at the front of this book where you will find instructions for getting our *Directory of Mail Order Pharmacies* and *Directory of Physicians*. These listings are updated monthly and, if there are any legal sources for GHB, you will find them there. (Please also read the 'Disclaimer' section at the front of this book.)

*"Shortly after I began taking L-dopa, I noticed that I had a stronger interest in sex and was thinking about it more frequently. Also, a low grade depression I had was alleviated. Incidently, my sex drive before L-dopa was pretty strong."*

—40-year-old man

# L-Dopa

***Prosexual uses of L-dopa:*** ─────────────────

| | |
|---|---|
| **Men:** | increased erectile capacity. |
| **Men & Women:** | enhanced subjective enjoyment of sex; increased libido; increased power and frequency of orgasm. |

In the popular and critically-acclaimed movie *Awakenings* (adapted from the bestselling book of the same name), actor/comedian Robin Williams brilliantly plays the role of pioneering physician and medical researcher Oliver Sacks. The film tells the true story of Sacks' efforts in the late 'sixties to assist survivors of an outbreak of *sleeping sickness* that had struck nearly five million people almost a half-century before. Many of these now quite elderly individuals had subsisted for decades in a zombie-like condition: they never went to sleep, and yet they never seemed fully awake.

*Awakenings* portrays the miracles and tragedies that followed when Sacks was able to rouse a small group of these patients from their fifty-year long trance. The catalyst for these astonishing transformations—or "awakenings"—was a drug just then entering widespread clinical use for Parkinson's disease. Similarities between some of the symptoms of Parkinson's and certain syndromes exhibited by his sleeping sickness patients had prompted Sacks to try out the new breakthrough drug—called L-dopa.

## What is L-Dopa?

Levodopa (L-3,4-dihydroxyphenylalanine) or L-dopa, for short, is found naturally in the human body (as well as in the bodies of other animals). It also occurs in some foods, including Velvet beans. L-dopa is an amino acid, an organic molecule incorporating an ammonia-like structure (or *amine*). Amino acids are the building blocks of proteins and of many neurochemicals. Because of its status as an amino acid and its natural presence in the body and in foods, L-dopa is sometimes called a nutrient in spite of its classification by the FDA as a prescription drug.

L-dopa is a precursor of dopamine. Like many other drugs that have come to be recognized for prosexual and life-extension properties, L-dopa was first widely used as a treatment for an aging-related syndrome—in this case, Parkinson's disease. (L-dopa has been the centerpiece of Parkinson's treatment for more than twenty-five years.)

## What Does It Do?

L-dopa is one is one of a series of *precursors* or building blocks used by the body to manufacture the neurotransmitters dopamine, norepinephrine, and epinephrine. It could be viewed as one link in a chain of several chemicals, each of which is converted by metabolic processes into the next.

This chain begins with the essential amino acid phenylalanine, found in the human diet. The body converts phenylalanine into tyrosine (also a dietary amino acid). Tyrosine is metabolized into dopa. (Please see the gray box below titled "Why is it called L-dopa?") Dopa is then converted into the neurotransmitter dopamine, some of which is then metabolized into the neurotransmitter norepinephrine. In turn, some of the norepinephrine produced is transformed into epinephrine (also a neurotransmitter).

As long as the metabolism is working fairly smoothly, *loading* the body with any of the precursors in this sequence—phenylalanine,

## Why is it called "L-dopa"?

The "L" in L-dopa stands for *levo*, which means left or left-hand. For this reason, some texts call it "levodopa," using the unabbreviated name for this substance. (This "L" has the same meaning as that often affixed to other nutrient amino acids, as in L-phenylalanine, L-tyrosine, and L-tryptophan.)

Chemical compounds usually appear in variant forms known as *isomers*, distinguished by their action on a ray of light. In this situation, the crystals formed by the molecules act like tiny prisms. A ray of light directed at the *levo-isomer* of a compound will be bent towards the left. A ray directed at the *dextro-isomer*, or right-hand variety, will be bent towards the right. ("Dexedrine," the name for a widely used stimulant and appetite suppressant, is short for "dextro-amphetamine," the right-hand isomer of amphetamine.) Some compounds also feature a *stereo-isomer* form, which will split the ray into two beams, one bent towards the left and the other towards the right.

A balanced mixture of dextro- and levo- isomers is known as a racemic mixture or *racemate*. Most routes of laboratory synthesis first produce racemates, from which one or the other isomer must then be isolated if desired.

Among compounds used as drugs, especially those considered psychoactive, one of the two isomers—almost always the levo-isomer—is usually significantly more active than the other. This is the case with L-dopa, the left hand form of the amino acid known as *dopa*. L-dopa's right-hand twin, *dextrodopa*, is relatively inactive and is therefore not marketed.

tyrosine, or dopa—will result in greater brain levels of norepinephrine. This loading can be accomplished through diet or supplementation.

Because dopa is the immediate precursor of dopamine, loading with L-dopa is a fast, direct, and efficient way to produce heightened dopamine levels in the brain. (Brain dopamine levels cannot be increased by administering dopamine directly because it does not cross the blood/brain barrier.)

**Biosynthesis of Dopamine, Norepinephrine, and Epinephrine**

By taking advantage of the body's pre-existing metabolic pathway for manufacturing neurotransmitters, L-dopa stimulates both the dopamine and the norepinephrine systems of the brain. These neurotransmitter systems play important roles in libido and sex function. For instance, as discussed in the chapter called "Some Basic Physiology," these chemical messengers energize the activity of the brain's *sex center*, found in the brain region known as the *hypothalamus*.

A corollary of L-dopa's augmentation of dopamine levels can be a reduction in cerebral serotonin levels [Ballivet, 1973]. This serotonin decrease may also serve a prosexual function [Laborit, 1972], as high levels of this *inhibitory* neurotransmitter in the hypothalamus can *dampen* the activity of the sex center. Like several other dopamine agonists, L-dopa is also a powerful enhancer of growth hormone levels and inhibitor of prolactin levels.

## L-Dopa & Parkinson's

Parkinson's Disease is associated with low levels of dopamine and with degeneration of the dopamine system in a part of the brain called the *substantia nigra*. This tiny region of the brain is an important center of dopamine manufacture and features the highest dopamine concentration anywhere in the nervous system [Dean, 1993]. The dopamine system plays a key role in body movement and motor control; thus, the decreased integrity of the dopamine system found in Parkinson's manifests as the shakiness, loss of motor control, and rigidity of the body easily observed in people suffering from this syndrome.

L-dopa was first introduced as a treatment for Parkinson's Disease in 1961 and since 1967 has been the mainstay of therapy for this condition [Barbeau, 1976]. By interceding in the metabolic pathway described earlier, L-dopa restores dopamine levels in Parkinson's patients, resulting in significant alleviation of symptoms.

A 1972 report of a long-term clinical trial involving 216 Parkinson's patients offered the following effusive evaluation of L-dopa therapy:

> *"It is abundantly clear that [L-dopa] is far more effective than any drug previously used for this common and often devastating disease. Experience has shown that side effects, though frequent, can be reduced to acceptable levels by careful administration of the drug and by frequent supervision of the patient's progress...the majority of patients in this study accepted the more distressing side effects of [L-dopa] with only little complaint, as they enjoyed a release from many, if not all of their previous disabilities."*
> [Selby, 1972].

As the decades have passed, however, it has become clear that L-dopa offers only symptomatic improvement in those suffering from Parkinson's Disease. It does not ultimately retard the progress of the disease, and its effectiveness usually begins to decline after five to seven years. These limitations are perhaps due to the fact that, while L-dopa increases dopamine levels, it does not address the damage to the dopamine neurons themselves that characterizes Parkinson's. Thus deprenyl, a compound which appears to feature advantages over L-dopa in several areas, may be on its way to replacing L-dopa as the mainstay of Parkinson's therapy [Dean, 1993]. (See the chapter on deprenyl for more information on its role in the treatment of Parkinson's.)

## Various Uses of L-dopa

Like most strongly prosexual compounds, L-dopa offers benefits in a wide range of other arenas. Aside from therapy for Parkinson's, uses for L-dopa include life extension, cognitive enhancement, weight loss, and protection against free radicals.

### Rejuvenation & life extension

L-dopa is mentioned quite frequently in Vladimir M. Dilman and Ward Dean's ground-breaking book, *The Neuroendocrine Theory of Aging and Degenerative Disease,* as a medication which may be capable of reversing—and even preventing—much of the deterioration associated with aging. Dilman and Dean emphasize L-dopa's ability to restore the sensitivity of the hypothalamus to feedback-inhibition, thereby assisting this region of the brain in its function of maintaining biochemical homeostasis within the body. (For further discussion of the hypothalamus and homeostasis, see the chapter entitled "Some Basic Physiology.") With regard to L-dopa's potential in life extension, they cite studies in which this compound restored menstrual cycling to post-menopausal female animals [Dilman, 1992]. (This effect is identical to that observed with bromocriptine both in animals and in some female human beings.)

*L-dopa guzzlers win mouse marathon.* In a well known experiment published in 1977, L-dopa was demonstrated to exert a significant life-extending effect in mice. This trial could almost be visualized as a life-extension marathon with four competing teams of mice: a control group fed no L-dopa; a second group given one milligram of L-dopa per gram of feed; a third group fed twenty milligrams of L-dopa per gram of feed; and a forth group consuming a whopping forty milligrams of L-dopa with every gram of feed.

At the three-hundred day point, the group fed one milligram of L-dopa per gram of diet had a better survival rate than any of the other groups. Oddly enough, this group nonetheless completely died out one hundred days before any of the other groups. The forty-milligram group—perhaps in part because these mice were given such a large dose without prior gradual upward titration—showed the highest initial mortality rate. However, at five hundred days, over eighty per cent of this group was still living—as compared to *less than fifty per cent* of the control group (fed no L-dopa). Thereafter, the forty milligram group maintained the highest survival rate until approximately the nine-hundred-fifty day point, when it was overtaken by the twenty-milligram group—a few members of which survived past the 1,000 day mark. (The control group was completely extinguished at approximately nine hundred and thirty days.) Overall, the "winning team"—the group maintaining the highest survival rate for the longest period of time—was clearly the forty milligram group [Cotzias, 1977].

*Aging rats perform swimmingly.* A striking demonstration of L-dopa's life extension capacities occurred in an experiment comparing the swimming ability of young adult rats with that of old rats both before and after the latter were given L-dopa. The swimming style of old rats without L-dopa characteristically featured inefficient posture and use of bodily movements, as well as a low level of endurance. After a fairly short time, these old rats would run out of steam and begin to sink.

However, after they were given L-dopa, the swimming performance of the older rats became indistinguishable from that of younger rats, showing the same level of stamina as well as efficient posture and use of body movement. This improvement no doubt reflects L-dopa's stimulation of the dopamine system, which plays a vital role in physical movement and coordination [Boyd, 1970].

### As a stimulant

L-dopa has gained a following as an all-purpose stimulant and aid to stamina, and as such has been a boon to some people desiring to increase the duration of their exercise and work-out periods [Pearson, 1982]. In these capacities its effects have been compared to those of amphetamine. However, at least at the dosage levels used for such purposes, L-dopa causes fewer side effects than amphetamines and less tension or edginess. L-dopa also lacks the unpleasant, sometimes depressive aftermath (known as the "crash") and is not addictive.

The comparison with amphetamines is not surprising, as L-dopa energizes precisely the same neurotransmitter systems. In fact, L-dopa is sometimes used as an amphetamine substitute or as a treatment for withdrawal symptoms in individuals attempting to kick an amphetamine addiction.

### Appetite suppression & weight loss

Like amphetamines, one of the effects of L-dopa is appetite suppression. This is one factor that can lead to weight loss with the use of L-dopa. Another factor is the stimulation of growth hormone release, which improves the ratio of lean muscle to fat. L-dopa has been successfully used by many for weight-loss purposes, but it apparently does not work well for truly obese individuals [Pearson, 1982].

### As an antioxidant

L-dopa is a powerful antioxidant [Pearson, 1982]. However, L-dopa itself *autoxidates*, or spontaneously oxidizes, into free-radical byproducts. Therefore, some experts recommend an increased intake of other antioxidants with the use of L-dopa. [Pearson, 1982]. (See the section below entitled "Oxidation & vitamin C.")

# L-Dopa & Sex

Data about the sexual effects of L-dopa comes from several major arenas. One of the most widely discussed is the history of "hypersexual" episodes among some of those being treated with L-dopa for Parkinsonism. Aside from these more extreme cases, L-dopa has a good track record for improving the sexual dysfunction and loss of libido often associated with Parkinson's. Additionally, there have been a number of experiments assessing the effects of L-dopa on the sexual behavior of animals. We also have collected a noteworthy body of anecdotal evidence for prosexual effects among normal and healthy individuals using L-dopa for experimental life extension purposes. And at least two of the possible mechanisms for L-dopa's prosexual effects—increase of dopamine and inhibition of pituitary prolactin release—have been studied and quantified.

Much of the research into L-dopa's sexual effects has concluded that supplementation with this compound enhances libido only in those whose L-dopa levels are low to begin with—a condition that would normally be accompanied by a low initial sex drive [Gawin, 1978]. This finding, however, is not entirely consistent with the anecdotal evidence from life-extension and smart drug circles, summarized below.

### "Hypersexuality" in Parkinson's patients

In all likelihood it was the appearance of a syndrome identified as "hypersexuality" among Parkinson's patients (especially males) being treated with L-dopa that first drew attention to the prosexual potential of this compound. ("Hypersexuality" refers to a level of interest in sex and sexual activity intense enough to be judged abnormal or unhealthy.) This phenomenon has been a subject of several medical papers [Uitti, 1989; Vogel, 1983; Buffum, 1982; Ballivet 1973].

Studies have reported the rate of hypersexual behavior among L-dopa-treated Parkinson's patients at as low as just under one percent [Buffum, 1982] and as high as eleven percent [Ballivet, 1973].

*Possible hidden factors in*
*Parkinsonian "hypersexuality"*

In attempting to understand reports of L-dopa-
induced "hypersexuality" among aging Parkinson's
patients, it may be important to critically assess
the overall context in which the label "hypersexual" was assigned.

The patients in question were not only elderly, but
suffered from a disease known to impair libido and
sexual function [Singer, 1992; Koller, 1990]. Any
eruption of intense interest in sex among such
individuals might be disturbing to others *merely*
*because of its utterly unexpected nature.*

The environments, whether domestic or clinical, in
which these surges of sexuality occurred were
adapted to the care of severely debilitated people
and were thus unprepared to provide constructive
outlets for strong sexual feelings. In such unready
environments, almost any overt sexual behavior
would probably have been perceived as disruptive.

Such factors could easily have encouraged the tendency—perhaps most pronounced in the psychiatric arena—of many medical practitioners to apply
pathological labels to any sufficiently disturbing or
disruptive behavior on the part of their patients. In
at least one relevant paper, simple "increased
libido" in Parkinson's patients was included among
side effects classified as psychiatric disturbances
[Girke, 1975]—whereas in other papers the same
phrase was used to indicate improvement [Brown,
1978]. Such discrepancies can easily be viewed as
evidence of the role of personal bias and cultural
*mores* in the theory and practice of medicine. In
another study, the operational definition of
"hypersexuality" involved not objective clinical
criteria, but rather "sexual behavior on treatment
[that] became of concern to the patient's family or

> a social agency" [Uitti, 1989].
>
> The point here is that what is "aberrant" is to some degree a matter of context and point of view. (Such differences in bias may been one underlying factor in the inability of the experts even to approach consensus on the origin of the behavior in question.) The abrupt appearance of a level of sexual enthusiasm that would be considered admirably normal and healthy for a young man in his late teens or early twenties could easily be dismissed as pathological in a different sociomedical context—for instance, that of a clinic for aging Parkinson's patients. Thus it seems possible that at least *some* of these cases of "hypersexuality," had they occurred in a different context, might instead have been hailed as the miraculous restoration of youthful sexual vigor to the previously aged and decrepit.

Different authors attribute this effect to widely divergent causes. One paper views it as part of a generalized L-dopa-initiated hypomanic syndrome [Buffum, 1982]. (Hypomania is the psychiatric term for a level of agitation and overstimulation short of that characterizing classic mania.) Another concludes that it is purely and simply a consequence of prolactin inhibition [Uitti, 1989]. Some sources insist that sexual behavior prior to treatment is the key determining factor [Buffum, 1982; Angrist, 1986], while, on a somewhat similar track, another group of authors characterize L-dopa's role in such cases as that of "unmasking...a latent sexual deviation in Parkinsonian patients" [Quinn, 1983].

### Sexual benefits in Parkinsonism

Loss of sex drive and various forms of sexual dysfunction, including problems with erection among over 60% of male patients, are common symptoms of Parkinson's disease [Singer, 1992; Koller,

1990; Bianchine, 1979]. L-dopa is effective in addressing these issues as well as the other problems associated with Parkinson's [Koller, 1990].

In one study of male Parkinsonian patients, about 50% of the men reported increased libido as a result of L-dopa treatment. This study concludes that L-dopa also improves sexual *function* in Parkinsonian men, given that certain key aspects of their endocrine function have not been damaged [Brown, 1978].

### Animal studies

Some scientists conducting animal experiments with L-dopa concluded that this compound increased libido in most of the animals observed [Buffum, 1982]. Overall results from animal studies on L-dopa's sexual effects, however, are much more ambiguous.

One report refers to the "lordosis-inhibiting action of...L-dopa" in female rats [Sietnieks, 1982]. Since *lordosis* is an arching of the spine understood as a sign of sexual receptivity, L-dopa would appear in this experiment to have exerted an anti-sexual effect. (This finding is consistent with a study discussed in the chapter on bromocriptine, in which lowered levels of prolactin apparently decreased lordosis behavior in female rats.)

Among studies of male rat sexual behavior we find conclusions of every possible variety: that L-dopa facilitates sexual behavior; that L-dopa inhibits such behavior; and that L-dopa has no significant effect in this area. One experiment with male rats who had previously shown a low level of sexual activity found L-dopa to have sexually stimulatory effects [Tagliamonte, 1974]. Conversely, in a study with "sexually vigorous" males, L-dopa exerted sexually inhibitory action [Gray, 1974]. Another experiment found that lower doses of L-dopa increased copulatory behavior, whereas higher doses decreased it [Malmas, 1976]. One study concluded that "sexual behavior was not altered by L-dopa" [Ryan, 1979], echoing an earlier experiment in which "L-dopa brought about no definite change in amount of time spent in overall sexual activity" [Keyes, 1976].

A number of factors may have played significant roles in producing the disparities among these results. Some of these experiments used castrated rats treated with testosterone—a fairly common technique in such experiments, the purpose of which is to minimize variability in the rats' testosterone levels.

Other experiments, however, used rats that were gonadally intact. Furthermore, the dosages of L-dopa used differed greatly from experiment to experiment; rats in some of the studies were *pre*-treated with various compounds; and in some cases, L-dopa was administered simultaneously with catalysts or synergists.

In spite of the sharp inconsistencies in the methodologies and results of animal experimentation with sexual behavior and L-dopa, it seems nonetheless widely accepted within the scientific community that this compound features a "stimulating action on sexuality" [Castaigne, 1975].

### Good news from life extension circles

L-dopa is mentioned by Durk Pearson and Sandy Shaw in *Life Extension* as an agent that increases brain levels of norepinephrine and dopamine, and may therefore "increase sexual interest and activity." As a compound that stimulates these neurotransmitter systems, facilitates growth hormone release, decreases prolactin levels, and reduces serotonin levels, L-dopa could reasonably be expected to charge both male and female libido, facilitate male erection, and perhaps even increase the power and frequency of orgasm for both sexes.

Nevertheless, aside from sexual effects on Parkinson's sufferers and a few groups of patients with serious psychiatric problems [Buffum, 1982], little if any scientific research has been performed to test L-dopa's prosexual potential. One exception is a study in which L-dopa increased the rate of spontaneous erection in six of eight men [Buffum, 1982].

Thus, as with GHB, most of the evidence for L-dopa's sexual efficacy—particularly among normal, healthy individuals—is anecdotal in nature. In recent years, L-dopa has developed a substantial following among those pursuing life extension and cognition enhancement. Within these circles, L-dopa has gained a significant reputation for increasing sex drive as well as enjoyment of sex. Dr. Ward Dean has mentioned that L-dopa and deprenyl are among the substances that he prescribes for life extension purposes that his patients consistently comment upon with regard to strong prosexual effects.

### Prolactin and growth hormone effects

The anti-sexual properties of high prolactin levels have been discussed at length in the chapter on bromocriptine. L-dopa, like bromocriptine, is an effective inhibitor of pituitary prolactin release. Five hundred milligrams of L-dopa will suppress prolactin levels for more than four hours. Suppression is greatest at around the three hour point, where prolactin levels drop to under forty percent of baseline levels [Dilman, 1992].

The same amount of L-dopa (five hundred milligrams) has been used to increase growth hormone output of healthy males in their 60s to levels approaching those characteristic of young adults. Pearson and Shaw recommend L-dopa supplementation as an aid to wound healing because of these powerful growth hormone effects [Pearson, 1982].

# L-Dopa, Oxidation & Vitamin C

Various researchers have suggested that at least some of the degradation of the brain's dopamine system characteristic of Parkinsonism is caused by oxidative free radical byproducts of dopamine. According to this scenario, increasing the brain's dopamine levels by administering L-dopa, while providing short-term relief of symptoms, could actually accelerate the course of the disease in the long run. This process might even be further aggravated by the presence of free-radicals occurring due to the oxidation of L-dopa itself. (The adjunctive use of bromocriptine with L-dopa for the purpose of minimizing—and perhaps even reversing—this damage has been discussed in the chapter on bromocriptine) [Pearson, 1982; Block, 1993].

Of course, concerns about such oxidative damage are not nearly as significant for those using L-dopa for prosexual or life extension purposes as for Parkinson's patients. The dosages used for life-extension and sex-enhancement are only a fraction of those required to treat Parkinsonism. Furthermore, most people embarking on a life-extension or sex-enhancement program employing L-dopa will not be suffering from the high level of prior oxidative damage to the dopamine system that is suspected to play a key role in Parkinsonism.

Nevertheless, preventing and minimizing free-radical damage—a primary contributor to the aging process and quite possibly to the decline of sexual function as well—should be a focus of attention for everyone concerned with sexual health and with well-being in general. For those using L-dopa, there is an easy and reliable means of addressing this issue: our venerable nutritional hero, vitamin C.

Vitamin C has been clearly demonstrated to prevent the spontaneous oxidation of L-dopa [Pearson, 1982]. Furthermore, it offers other equally important benefits for those using L-dopa. Vitamin C plays a significant assisting role in the synthesis of catecholamines—the class of neurotransmitters to which dopamine and norepinephrine belong—and in maintaining levels of these chemicals in the body. Because of these properties, vitamin C should help make the action of catecholamine precursors like L-dopa more efficient, reducing the dosage required by offering more dopamine for your L-dopa dollars. In research with Parkinson's patients, four grams of vitamin C on a daily basis allowed a two-gram reduction of daily L-dopa intake without loss of treatment efficacy [Pearson, 1982]. In sum, vitamin C offers a nearly ideal catalyst/synergist, or biochemical partner, for L-dopa.

While vitamin C prevents the oxidation of L-dopa itself, other antioxidants may be required to combat oxidation of the dopamine into which L-dopa is converted. In *Life Extension*, Durk Pearson and Sandy Shaw recommend any or all of the following antioxidants for preventing damage to the dopamine system by oxidative dopamine byproducts: Hydergine, vitamins E, B-1, B-5, and B-6, and minerals zinc and selenium [Pearson, 1982]. (For a discussion of the possible complications involved in using B-6 in conjunction with L-dopa, please see the section below entitled "The vitamin B-6 issue.")

### Carbidopa

L-dopa is converted into dopamine by an enzyme called *decarboxylase*; this process is therefore called *decarboxylation*. This conversion occurs both within the brain and in peripheral tissue. In fact, the lion's share of any given dose of L-dopa taken orally undergoes decarboxylation *before* it reaches the brain. The dopamine thus produced is unavailable to the brain—where it is needed for therapeutic and prosexual effects—because it cannot cross the blood-brain barrier.

The resultant increase of dopamine concentrations in peripheral tissue serves little purpose, and may merely aggravate side effects, particularly nausea and vomiting. This phenomenon also requires that a much larger quantity of L-dopa be administered than would be necessary if a greater portion were able to reach the brain prior to decarboxylation.

The solution to this problem represents a brilliant example of pharmacological synergy. Carbidopa is a compound that inhibits the action of decarboxylase, preventing the conversion of L-dopa into dopamine. It performs this function *in peripheral tissue only* because carbidopa, unlike L-dopa itself, *does not cross the blood-brain barrier*. The simultaneous administration of carbidopa with L-dopa thus preserves L-dopa in the molecular form in which it is administered, making more of the amino acid available to cross into the brain where conversion into dopamine can then occur unimpeded.

Carbidopa has been shown to reduce the L-dopa requirements of Parkinson's patients by about *seventy-five percent*. It reduces the incidence of nausea and vomiting among Parkinson's patients, often allows dosages to be increased more rapidly to therapeutic levels once treatment has begun, and may result in a smoother response to treatment than L-dopa alone. Some Parkinson's patients who have not responded well to L-dopa by itself have been able to achieve successful treatment with L-dopa in combination with carbidopa. Studies with animals also suggest that carbidopa may prevent the heart arrhythmias that can sometimes occur as a side effect of L-dopa treatment (by preventing the increase of dopamine concentrations in heart tissue). Furthermore, carbidopa prolongs the action of L-dopa

[PDR, 1994; Fowkes, 1994].

L-dopa marketed under the brand name Sinemet contains both L-dopa and carbidopa in either a ten-to-one or a four-to-one mixture.

### The vitamin B-6 issue

Vitamin B-6 facilitates the decarboxylation of L-dopa both in the brain and in peripheral tissue. Because of this property, B-6 supplements taken by Parkinson's patients treated with L-dopa alone (that is, without carbidopa) have sometimes reversed the effects of L-dopa, leading to an increase in Parkinsonian symptoms. (Durk Pearson and Sandy Shaw, however, report that people *without* Parkinson's have successfully used small quantities of L-dopa for growth hormone and fat-loss purposes while continuing to supplement heavily with B-6.) [PDR, 1994; Pearson, 1982].

Carbidopa inhibits this action of B-6 in peripheral tissue. As mentioned earlier, B-6 is one of the antioxidants recommended for protecting the dopamine system against oxidative dopamine byproducts—levels of which are likely to increase with the use of a dopamine precursor such as L-dopa. For those who wish to use B-6 concurrently with L-dopa for this or other reasons, Sinemet—the form of L-dopa containing carbidopa—once again offers itself as the most attractive option.

## Precautions, Side Effects, & Contraindications

The following description of side effects and contraindications associated with L-dopa may seem rather serious and extensive. However, it is important to remember the context from which most of this information is derived: the treatment of Parkinson's disease. The vast majority of cases from which these risk-related data are drawn were elderly, already seriously ill, and were using L-dopa in dosages as high as eight grams per day—*sixteen times greater than the highest dose that might be used by a healthy individual seeking personal enhancement.* As for the levels of L-dopa commonly used for life extension, smart drug, and prosexual purposes, gerontologist Ward Dean has said: "These small doses greatly reduce the likelihood of occurrence of any serious adverse effects. I have never noted any such effects in my patients on these low doses" [Dean, 1993].

The inventory of possible negative reactions that follows is intended, therefore, not to alarm, but merely to inform—and to insure that the full spectrum of this compound's potential effects is presented in a balanced manner.

### Side effects & adverse reactions

The most common side effect of L-dopa is nausea, sometimes accompanied by vomiting. These effects occur even with the relatively small dosages used for life extension and prosexual purposes, but tend to disappear within the first few weeks of use. Irritability and insomnia can also occur at low doses, but also tend to be highly transient. Some appetite suppression is also common, and is more likely to persist. Headache may also occur. These effects result not from toxicity on the part of L-dopa itself but from stimulation of the dopamine system [Dean, 1993; Pearson, 1982; PDR, 1994]. (Techniques for minimizing or avoiding such effects are discussed below under "Dosage & Timing.")

The following possible side effects have also been observed, but *almost exclusively in cases of Parkinsonism and with higher dosages*: choreiform or dystonic movements (small involuntary body motions); conversely, bradykinetic episodes (slowing or decrease of body movement); orthostatic hypotension (a sharp drop in blood pressure upon suddenly standing up, experienced as dizziness); high blood pressure; heart palpitations and irregularity or slowing of the heartbeat; confusion, sleepiness, psychotic episodes, anxiety, agitation, overstimulation, or depression—sometimes accompanied by suicidal tendencies; gastrointestinal bleeding; duodenal ulcers; anemia; ataxia (discoordination); numbness; hand tremors, muscle twitching, and muscle spasms [Dean, 1993; Pearson, 1982; PDR, 1994].

### Contraindications & drug combinations

Those with pre-existing pigmented malignant melanomas, whose growth may be accelerated by the use of this compound, should not take L-dopa [Pearson, 1982; PDR, 1994]. L-dopa is contraindicated in those with wide-angle glaucoma. L-dopa may aggravate conditions of mania and schizophrenia.

Those using MAO inhibitors—with the exception of deprenyl—should avoid L-dopa in order to prevent possible severe hypertensive episodes. Except with forms of L-dopa containing carbidopa (marketed as Sinemet), vitamin B-6 supplements should not be used by Parkinson's patients being treated with L-dopa unless the physician has directed otherwise. Adverse reactions have occasionally been seen among those using tricyclic antidepressants with L-dopa, and neuroleptics (major tranquilizers) are likely to decrease the efficacy of L-dopa [Dean, 1993; Pearson, 1982; PDR, 1994].

(Further information regarding side effects and contraindications can be found by consulting entries in *The Physicians' Desk Reference* for Dopar, Larodopa, and Sinemet.)

## Dosage & Timing

As with other dopaminergics, it is generally advisable to slowly increase or *titrate* the dosage of L-dopa over several days until a desirable level of effect is achieved. Such an approach will usually bypass unwanted side-effects. If side effects do occur, a decrease in dosage will usually result in their rapid disappearance, and can be followed, if necessary, by even more gradual upward titration.

Dosages used for growth hormone release and fat loss, or for smart drug or experimental life extension purposes, are usually in the range of 125 to 500 milligrams daily [Dean, 1993; Pearson, 1982], either all at once or in two divided doses. This may also be an appropriate range for those seeking prosexual effects. Theoretically, those using L-dopa in conjunction with carbidopa may be able to achieve similar results with as little as 35 to 125 milligrams daily. Concentrating most or all of one's daily intake just prior to sleep is likely to maximize the benefits of L-dopa for those primarily interested in stimulating growth hormone release.

Those seeking cognition enhancement or stimulant effects should bear in mind that the level of L-dopa in the body usually reaches a peak within a half hour to two hours following ingestion, and begins to drop off one to three hours thereafter [Dean, 1993]. (The addition of carbidopa, as in Sinemet, will, as mentioned, prolong the effects of L-dopa.)

Sinemet is available in three mixtures: tablets containing 10 milligrams of carbidopa with 100 milligrams of L-dopa; tablets containing 25 milligrams of carbidopa with 100 milligrams of L-dopa; and tablets containing 25 milligrams of carbidopa with 250 milligrams of L-dopa. Sustained-release Sinemet is also available (under the brand name Sinemet CR) in two formulas, one containing 25 milligrams of carbidopa with 100 milligrams of L-dopa and the other containing 50 milligrams of carbidopa with 200 milligrams of L-dopa.

## Legality & Availability

L-dopa is available by prescription in the United States under the brand names Larodopa, Dopar, and Sinemet. L-dopa can also be obtained legally—without a prescription—from various overseas mail-order sources, as long as the quantity you order can reasonably be considered no more than a three-month personal supply. (Please note, however, that we still recommend you work with your personal physician.)

## Physicians and Product Sources

Please note the tearout card at the front of this book where you will find instructions for getting our *Directory of Mail Order Pharmacies* and *Directory of Physicians*. These listings are updated monthly. (Please also read the 'Disclaimer' section at the front of this book.)

*"Now I have a sex life again. And the sexual experience itself is better. Yohimbe has given me all this pleasure. I'm really glad I got into it."*

—71-year-old male

# Yohimbe & Yohimbine

## *Prosexual uses of yohimbe & yohimbine:* ———

Men: increased libido; ease, duration, & fullness of erection; spontaneous erection; more powerful orgasm; multiple orgasms & ejaculations; more forceful ejaculations; greater quantity of ejaculate; increased libido.

Women: insufficient data (see the section below called, "What About Women?")

## What are Yohimbe & Yohimbine?

*Corynanthe yohimbe* is the botanical name for a tree that grows in West Africa. For centuries—perhaps millennia—the folk medicine practiced by tribes in this region and the nearby West Indies islands has included a tea distilled from the inner bark of this tree. The brew is used to amplify male virility and sexual prowess. It is the traditional fuel for intense tribal sex ceremonies reported to last as long as half a month—rituals which might never have been possible but for the power of this concoction [Watson, 1993; Stafford, 1992; Griffin 1991; Gottlieb, 1974].

### Yohimbe vs. Yohimbine

A large selection of *Corynanthe* bark extracts, in both capsule and tincture forms, is widely available over-the-counter from health-food stores and other outlets for herbal supplements. These products are usually referred to simply as "yohimbe." *Yohimbine hydrochloride*—or "yohimbine"—has been isolated as the most active chemical compound in yohimbe bark, and has recently become available by prescription in the United States. Yohimbine is present in significant quantities in almost all of the over-the-counter herbal yohimbe products [Griffin, 1991].

### It's not just for impotence anymore

Current scientific and medical literature offers a rather limited portrayal of yohimbine's sexual properties in human beings that focuses almost exclusively on the treatment of male impotence. These discussions leave untouched the broad range of intense prosexual effects widely reported by men who have no sexual dysfunction at all. An impressive body of anecdotal evidence surrounds the use of yohimbe and yohimbine for making *good* sex even *better*.

"...One of the most popular aphrodisiac herbs available, yohimbe has a reputation for producing electrifying sexual encounters."
—Cynthia Watson M.D.
*Love Potions*

The stories of men who use these substances to push the envelope of sexual pleasure for themselves and their partners—often achieving spectacular results—are sampled in the section entitled "Yohimbe and Yohimbine for Sexual Excellence." Furthermore, animal studies and a tiny smattering of anecdotal reports suggest that yohimbe and yohimbine may hold prosexual potential for women as well as men. This issue is explored in the section entitled, "What About Women?"

### A twisted history

The recent history of yohimbe and yohimbine has followed a contorted path marked by confusion and reversal. A prescription impotence pill called "Afrodex" containing small quantities of yohimbine and other compounds was withdrawn from the American market in 1973 due to controversy about efficacy and safety [Rosen, 1993]. In the '60s, '70s, and early '80s, the existing literature on yohimbine often acknowledged that it could facilitate erection, but usually claimed that it had no impact on libido [Gawin, 1978]. These sources stated that yohimbine was therefore definitely *not* a real aphrodisiac. Such pronouncements persisted until a widely acclaimed animal study published in 1984 provided strong evidence that yohimbine stimulates libido (at least in male rats) and thereby qualifies as a "true aphrodisiac" [Clark, 1984].

The next few years saw the publication of a series of studies concerning yohimbine's efficacy in treating male impotence [Sonda, 1990; Susset, 1989; Reid, 1987; Morales, 1987]. FDA approval for this indication soon followed, and, after a twenty year absence, yohimbine reappeared on the roster of drugs that could be dispensed legally by prescription. Perhaps the most historically significant aspect of these events

> "In the past decade, there has been a marked resurgence of interest in yohimbine following a number of reports of prosexual effects in animal and human studies."
> —Rosen and Ashton
> *Prosexual Drugs ...*

was the appearance in the *Physicians' Desk Reference* of the following words: "It may have activity as an aphrodisiac" [PDR, 1994]. However tentatively phrased, this sentence is almost surely the first appearance of the term "aphrodisiac" in any edition of the *PDR*—which lists only those indications for a drug that have been sanctioned by the FDA—as well as its first use for decades in information released officially by a pharmaceutical firm.

The second coming of prescription yohimbine became an

opportunity for many physicians and medical authorities to warn the public against purchasing over-the-counter herbal yohimbe products (which had remained available during the decades of yohimbine's absence from approved medicine). These cautions were issued on the basis that the herbal alternatives supposedly featured so little—if any—yohimbine hydrochloride as to offer no possibility of therapeutic benefit.

The technical director of the U.S. Food and Dairy Labs performed a chemical analysis of ten different mail-order brands, expecting the results to prove this claim definitively. However, *all* of the samples turned out to contain significant quantities of yohimbine hydrochloride. In fact, *most* of these brands featured *more* yohimbine per capsule than the 5.4 milligrams contained in one prescription tablet. Better yet, in terms of cost per unit of yohimbine, many of the herbal extracts offered a *better deal* than the pharmaceutical products [Griffin, 1991].

Now that both yohimbine and its herbal antecedents have emerged from this checkered history with their value firmly established, these chemical "comeback kids" are doubtless here to stay. And although herbal preparations containing this compound have a long history of traditional use in other cultures, yohimbine has so recently appeared in modern medical practice that, as far as contemporary Western society is concerned, it is considered a *new* prosexual drug.

> "Yohimbine is the only substance with a specific FDA-approved indication as an aphrodisiac."
> —Ward Dean, M.D.

## How Does It Work?

Yohimbine's primary path of action—which is completely different from the other pharmacological mechanisms described in this book—duplicates a biochemical event believed to play a key role in producing male erection.

Yohimbine acts upon a very specific network of nerve cells

called the *alpha-2 adrenergic* system (a subsystem of the larger *adrenergic* system, so named because its functions are closely tied to the hormone adrenaline). Yohimbine effectively shuts down the alpha-2 adrenergic system by blocking receptor sites for the neurotransmitters that stimulate its activity. This blockade could be compared to putting tape over a light-switch to prevent the lights from being turned off.

Research has indicated that a natural alpha-2 adrenergic blockade performed by the body's own chemicals is part of the normal physiology of erection. According to theory, inhibition of the alpha-2 adrenergic system should increase the flow of blood through arteries into the penis, while at the same time decreasing the flow of blood out from the penis through veins. It may also result in higher levels of acetylcholine, a neurotransmitter closely associated with male erection [PDR, 1994; Adaikan, 1988].

In addition to promoting erection, yohimbine's blockade of alpha-2 adrenergic receptors is probably the central means by which this compound stimulates sex drive. Recent research has produced growing evidence that the adrenergic system affected by yohimbine is a critical factor in libido and sexual behavior [Clark, 1991; Clark, 1985; Clark, 1984; Smith, 1987A].

Further explanation for yohimbine's prosexual properties comes from a recent study with humans showing that this compound increases blood levels of the neurotransmitter norepinephrine by 66% [Grossman, 1993]. Norepinephrine stimulates the brain's sex center in the hypothalamus (see the chapter entitled "Some Basic Physiology") and, as discussed elsewhere in this book, is usually considered one of the body's natural prosexual chemicals. (Ironi-

The inventory manager of a large retail health-supplement outlet in Santa Cruz, California claims that the demand for yohimbe products has increased exponentially in the last year alone. "It's amazing," he says. "All of a sudden they're just flying off the shelf. New customers come in to ask about them every day. Lately, it's been hard for me to keep them in stock."

cally, yohimbine was formerly believed to *inhibit* release of norepinephrine [Yates, 1991].)

Surprisingly, animal studies have demonstrated that the heightened sex drive induced by yohimbine does *not* involve an increase in testosterone levels [Naumenko, 1991]. Furthermore, this compound stimulates sexual activity in castrated male rats with negligible testosterone, as well as in female rats during the *non-receptive* stage of their sexual cycle (when testosterone levels are quite low) [Clark, 1985]. Apparently, yohimbine's libido-enhancing power is *quite* independent of this hormone, which is commonly attributed with a crucial role in sexual motivation.

### Other possible mechanisms of action

Certain other mechanisms of action are consistently attributed to yohimbine in older popular literature covering this compound. No references to these effects appear in the extensive selection of recent scientific papers on yohimbine that have been reviewed in the research for this chapter. We have therefore devoted only the following brief summaries to these possible routes of action.

We have encountered several claims that yohimbine's erectile effects involve the spinal ganglia, nerve clusters that appear in rows just outside the spine on both the right and left sides. According to these sources, yohimbine stimulates the specific spinal ganglia that control male erection [Stafford, 1993; Miller, 1985; Gottlieb, 1974].

Some sources attribute a mild serotonin-inhibiting action to yohimbine [Gottlieb, 1974; Miller, 1985]. A positive impact on libido could also be expected from this effect. Serotonin has been mentioned many times in this book as a neurotransmitter credited with a dampening effect on sex drive and sex function. In many experiments, drugs that reduce serotonin levels have been demonstrated to stimulate sexual activity in animals [Laborit, 1972], while the sex-negative effects of Prozac and other popular serotonin-enhancing prescription drugs are now becoming well-known.

At least two popular books first published in the 'seventies describe yohimbine as an MAO inhibitor and recommend that the standard dietary restrictions applying to MAO inhibitors be followed when yohimbine or yohimbe extracts are used [Stafford, 1993;

Gottlieb, 1974]. (MAO inhibition has been explained in the chapter on deprenyl.) Additionally, several individuals who provided personal anecdotes for this book had apparently received similar information from one source or another.

However, we have found no mention of MAO inhibition in scientific papers on the action of yohimbine. Furthermore, the *Physicians' Desk Reference*, which provides extensive safety information with each entry, does not make reference to the dietary guidelines for MAO inhibitors in any of the entries dealing with yohimbine [PDR, 1994]. Given these facts, it is safe to conclude either that yohimbine *does not* in fact inhibit MAO, or that its MAO-inhibiting action is too minimal to warrant concern.

## Rats Revisited

In several experiments conducted by various researchers, yohimbine has consistently produced an impressive acceleration of sexual activity in male rats [Bowes, 1992; Sala, 1990; Smith, 1987A; Smith, 1987B; Clark, 1984]. Perhaps the most remarkable finding from these studies occurred when yohimbine stimulated mating behavior in rats that had previously displayed *no sexual activity at all* [Clark, 1984]. Yohimbine also increased the percentage of sexually inexperienced male rats able to achieve ejaculation in their first sexual encounter with a female—thereby meeting researchers' criteria for successful completion of the mating act.

As mentioned earlier, it was believed until fairly recently that yohimbine did *not* stimulate sex drive. Oddly enough, scientists maintained this conclusion even though yohimbine had *already* been shown to facilitate sexual behavior among animals. This effect, however, was attributed not to increased sex drive, but instead to one of two other factors. It was seen either as one manifestation of a generalized behavioral stimulation that was not *specifically* sexual in nature, or as a *response* to the penile erections induced by yohimbine.

Most of this reluctance to assign libidogenic qualities to yohimbine probably stemmed from the fact that no role in sexual motivation had yet been attributed to the alpha-adrenergic system—the primary target of this compound's pharmacological action. In fact, recognition of this physiological system's significance to sex drive resulted to a great extent from the unambiguous manner in which yohimbine's libido-enhancing power was demonstrated by the particular animal studies about to be discussed.

In two of these studies, researchers anesthetized the genitalia of some of the male rats being treated with yohimbine. Minimizing the rats' physical awareness of their own penises in this manner, it was reasoned, would largely factor out initiation of copulation triggered exclusively by yohimbine-induced erections. Any *significant* increase in sexual activity would then have to be attributed to amplified sex drive. In both experiments making use of this technique, the rats in question displayed "mounting behavior" with much greater frequency than usual—despite the numbness of their sexual apparatus [Smith, 1987A; Clark, 1984].

A study conducted in 1992 carefully tested the theory that yohimbine heightens sexual behavior in animals only as part of an overall stimulation of physical activity. First, the researchers classified rat behavior into several categories. Then, after giving the rats a dose of yohimbine already known to facilitate sexual behavior, they recorded changes in levels of activity within each of these categories.

Ironically, this known prosexual dose of yohimbine produced a general *reduction* of (non-sexual) activity among these rats. Yohimbine's facilitation of sexual behavior in male rats clearly could no longer be blamed on a global stimulatory effect.

### Crocodile lust

A controlled study conducted in San Diego confirmed that yohimbine's prosexual effects extend to reptiles. Eighteen male Nile crocodiles of the same age were placed in three groups among a total of ninety female crocodiles. Eight of the males were given two doses of yohimbine per day for the first week only of a three-month observation period.

A sort of sexual daylight savings time effect occurred during the week that yohimbine was administered. For this period of time only, the daily peak in sexual activity among treated animals began and ended one hour earlier.

Surprisingly, frequency of copulation was *not* greater among yohimbine-fuelled crocodiles. However, the frequency in this group of certain body movements specifically associated with mating *was* significantly higher.

The total cycle of mating activity lasted *three weeks longer* among crocodiles given yohimbine than among less fortunate reptiles deprived of this compound. This result means that *prosexual effects from yohimbine persisted for a minimum of eleven weeks after administration was discontinued.*

Lastly, *a significantly greater percentage of fertility occurred in eggs produced by females who had been mating with yohimbine-treated males*. This difference could not be attributed to more frequent copulation because, as mentioned earlier, yohimbine-treated males did *not* mate more often than controls. Therefore, in order to explain this phenomenon, researchers concluded that crocodiles probably had "more successful copulations" as a result of yohimbine [Morpurgo, 1992].

## Yohimbine & Impotence

Several controlled trials have been conducted to test the efficacy of yohimbine in treating impotence. In these studies, the proportion of men showing a positive response to yohimbine therapy has consistently fallen in the range of thirty-three to forty-six percent [Rosen, 1993; Sonda, 1990; Susset, 1989; Morales, 1987; Reid, 1987].

The phrase "positive response" does not necessarily indicate a *complete* disappearance of problems with erection. For instance, in one study reporting an overall positive response rate of thirty-four percent, "full and sustained erections" re-appeared among only *fourteen percent* of the men. Twenty percent more nonetheless experi-

Yohimbine therapy usually takes two to three weeks to exert its full effect [Susset, 1989].

enced some degree of improvement. And in a group of 215 men undergoing yohimbine therapy, thirty eight-percent experienced some benefit, but only five percent were "completely satisfied" [Susset, 1989].

This level of success has qualified yohimbine as an impotence treatment of only "modest effectiveness" [Morales, 1987]. However, it is important to remember that impotence occurs for a variety of reasons; it would be unrealistic to expect one substance to be universally effective. Given the low incidence of adverse reactions and the drawbacks of some other options (for instance, surgical implants and drugs that must be injected into the penis), yohimbine has been recommended as the "first line of treatment" for this problem [Susset, 1989; Morales, 1987].

### For whom does it work best?

The studies discussed above produced some interesting results regarding yohimbine's varying success rates among different groups of patients. In one study, for instance, yohimbine demonstrated much greater efficacy for relatively mild, short-term problems with erection than for longer-lasting, more severe cases [Rosen, 1993; Susset, 1989].

"Most patients with changes in erectile response also reported increased sexual desire, and 4 out of 11 patients reported improved orgasm on yohimbine" [Rosen, 1993].

A more surprising finding occurred when researchers compared yohimbine's relative success in treating the two major diagnostic categories of impotence: *psychogenic* impotence, which results from psychological issues; and *organic* impotence, which can be traced to an underlying medical problem. Treatment approaches for these two types are usually very different.

Quite unexpectedly, yohimbine produced the *same* overall response rate in *both* categories. In fact, yohimbine's level of success for psychogenic impotence was roughly equal to that of sex therapy and marital counseling—two commonly recommended approaches to this type of problem [Morales, 1987].

The *Physicians' Desk Reference* specifically indicates yohimbine in cases of impotence with "psychogenic, vascular, or diabetic origins" [PDR, 1994].

## Yohimbine & Age-Related Male Sexual Decline

One experiment was performed specifically to find out whether yohimbe could restore the flagging libidos of aging male rats. The researchers reported that yohimbine increased the rate of sexual activity in a group of such animals according to all of the criteria used for measurement. In fact, the older rats reached a level of sexual vigor comparable to that observed in a group of much younger males. Neither of these groups, however, managed to match the pace of a third team benefitting from the combined advantages of both youth *and* yohimbine [Smith, 1990].

Elderly men suffering from chronic problems with erection participated in a month-long controlled study using relatively high doses of yohimbine. Thirty-four percent of the those given yohimbine experienced improvement, as compared to only five percent of those given placebo. This response rate falls well within the range reported by other impotence studies with yohimbine. However, the patients in this trial were advanced in age and featured a particularly high incidence of medical conditions that can interfere with male potency. Given these factors, researchers found the response rate of thirty-four percent "encouraging."

Furthermore, although many medications cause a greater frequency of side effects among the aged, the fairly high doses of yohimbine used here produced "only a few and benign side effects" among the elderly men who participated [Susset, 1989].

## Countering the Negative Sexual Effects of Other Medications

An article in the November, 1994 issue of *Penthouse* documents the hidden damage to many sex lives that has been caused by a variety of over-the-counter and prescription drugs. Yohimbine may offer help for those suffering from the sexual problems that can result from certain commonly-used medications.

### Antidepressants

Prozac is a member of a fairly new class of drugs called *serotonin reuptake blockers*. These compounds, used widely in recent years for treating depression and compulsive behavior, have become increasingly associated with difficulty achieving orgasm, problems with erection, and loss of libido.

In one survey of 160 people for whom Prozac had successfully alleviated depression, *thirty-four percent* reported problems with sexual function that began after they started taking Prozac. Nine of these people participated in a study investigating yohimbine's ability to reverse these effects. *Eight of the nine* reported improvement in response to a fairly moderate dose of yohimbine, although two stopped taking it because of side effects [Jacobsen, 1992].

A similar study involved six patients experiencing decreased sexual function as a result of serotonin reuptake blockers. *Five of the six* responded positively to individually-tailored doses of yohimbine

"Nearly 200 drugs on today's market have a direct impact on sexuality. The pills can leave men impotent, libidoless...50 to 75 percent of all sexual problems can be traced to a physical cause. In one out of four cases, the culprit is a pill...Drug companies testing new products don't spend time sleuthing out sexual pitfalls, and they rarely provide detailed data about what their drugs do in the bedroom...The most common sexual offenders are high-blood-pressure medications—including beta blockers, diuretics, and other drugs—which research shows can cause impotence or sexual malfunction in up to 70 percent or more of the men who take them."

—Amy Linn
*Penthouse* magazine, November 1994

[Hollander, 1992]. (The one exception, it should be noted, "failed to comply with yohimbine treatment.")

Both of these studies were *open trials*—meaning that they did not include a control group—and involved relatively small numbers of people. However, the evidence obtained was deemed sufficiently positive to warrant the conclusion that "yohimbine may be an effective treatment for the sexual side effects caused by serotonin reuptake blockers" [Hollander, 1992].

Clomipramine, an entirely different type of antidepressant, is frequently associated with inability to achieve orgasm. A report in a medical journal describes a case in which yohimbine was used successfully to alleviate this problem [Price, 1990].

### Animal studies with clonidine

Several animal studies have involved both yohimbine and clonidine, a drug used to control high blood pressure. This compound can result in impotence and loss of libido in human beings [PDR, 1994].

Researchers have found that clonidine can interfere with the sexual function of animals in several ways. (Some of these effects take place only when the drug is injected into certain arteries or brain regions; the normal use of clonidine in human beings will not necessarily produce the same results.) In dogs, clonidine can be used to reduce blood flow to the penis, and can decrease the size of ejaculations. In male rats, it can suppress sexual activity, and can prevent ejaculation entirely. In female rats, it can inhibit sexually receptive behavior.

Yohimbine blocks *all* of these clonidine-induced effects in animals [Yonezawa 1992; Clark, 1991; Clark, 1985; Davis 1977].


## Yohimbe & Yohimbine for Sexual Excellence

Yohimbe and yohimbine may well produce their most impressive and consistent prosexual effects among those who are already sexually healthy to begin with. In fact, it appears that growing numbers of men are using these substances for purposes of sex-enhancement as opposed to the treatment of any specific sexual dysfunction.

They report the following results: heightened libido; increased tactile sensation in the genitals and other parts of the body; longer, harder, larger erections; phenomenal stamina; more powerful orgasms; multiple orgasms and ejaculations; and greater quantity of ejaculate.

In at least some men, yohimbine can induce spontaneous erections even when sexual stimulation is absent. In one study, yohimbine demonstrated this capacity in twenty percent of the men used as test subjects [Buffum, 1985]. Several of the men interviewed for this book have experienced this phenomenon with herbal yohimbe products. In fact, some of them *always* have spontaneous erections when they use these substances. This effect generally seems to take place in the range of twenty minutes to an hour after ingestion.

One thirty-year old man first tried yohimbe by using the traditional technique of boiling the bark of the *yohimbehe* tree to produce a tea. An hour after drinking this extract, he was riding his bicycle. "I'd completely forgotten about the yohimbe," he says. "I was just riding merrily along, enjoying the weather, when suddenly I got this *huge* erection. I was totally flabbergasted. I hadn't even

"I started using yohimbe about three years ago, when I was sixty-eight. For a few years before that, I had been hesitant to pursue sexual relationships. I was really afraid of AIDS and other STDs, so for quite some time I abstained—even from safe sex—because I thought perhaps it was too risky. I kind of lost interest and didn't pursue it, although my sex drive was still present.

"When I started taking yohimbe, it sharply increased my libido right away. This effect was so strong that it overrode the inhibitions I had developed, and I started looking for partners again. I became more confident, more assertive, and more self-aware in the way I approached prospective sexual partners."

—71-year-old male

been thinking about sex! Then I remembered the yohimbe. Wow!"

One man in his fifties consistently gets spontaneous erections from yohimbe. He describes "extraordinarily large erections of maximum length and angle that usually last for two or three hours."

This man also claims that yohimbe "returns my youthful capacity for multiple ejaculations. And I don't lose my erection between orgasms. I produce much more ejaculate, and my ejaculations are *very* forceful; they actually travel a couple of feet."

Most men who use yohimbe or yohimbine for sex-enhancement purposes take these substances intermittently to obtain short-term effects for appropriate occasions. One exception is a twenty-nine year-old video-store owner interviewed for this book.

This man first heard about yohimbine from associates in the X-rated film business. "I tried it out," he says. "It was the best thing that ever happened. I swear by that. I had longer, thicker, longer-lasting erections and bigger ejaculations, and the feeling that it gives you is incredible."

Although he had never experienced any problems with erection, he began using yohimbine on a daily basis, a prac-

More than one source interviewed for this book mentioned that yohimbe and yohimbine serve as "tools of the trade" for many actors in the X-rated film industry, who use them to meet the rigorous demands of their profession.

tice he has maintained for about two years. Over this time period, he has "turned on around twenty male friends" to yohimbine hydrochloride. All of them are relatively young and in good sexual health. Most of these men now also use yohimbine every day, in dosages that vary according to their anticipated of level of sexual activity.

"I've not found one person who's tried it," claims the video store owner, "that didn't have a positive sexual response."

## Yohimbine's Subjective Effects

A guide to herbal therapies for men claims that yohimbe promotes "increased sense of well being and a sense of openness" [Green, 1991]. One middle-aged man interviewed for this book says that his use of yohimbe tinctures sometimes produces "a mild, enjoyable feeling of stimulation."

Higher doses of yohimbe can be accompanied by mildly "psychedelic" effects lasting a few hours [Stafford, 1993; Watson, 1993; Miller, 1985; Gottlieb, 1974]. These phenomena have been characterized as "a general sensory intensification" or "hyperaesthesia" [Gawin, 1978]. *Sex Drugs and Aphrodisiacs* by Adam Gottlieb describes the following sensations:

> "...*warm spinal shivers, which are especially enjoyable during coitus and orgasm (bodies feel like they are melting into one another), psychic stimulations, mild perceptual changes without hallucination, and heightening of emotional and sexual feeling.*" [Gottlieb, 1974]

The young video store owner quoted at length in the section on "Yohimbe and Yohimbine for Sexual Excellence" has occasionally obtained "something of a high" from prescription yohimbine (which he sometimes takes in unusually large doses). He describes this experience in terms of "a strong mental effect. I tend to get a little discombobulated, but somehow still feel *more* mentally alert. Sometimes I get little body shakes. I like these feelings; they don't interfere with sleep, and they seem very natural."

Our research has yielded only a few accounts of markedly psychoactive effects resulting from the use of yohimbine or preparations containing it. Fairly standard dosages of these substances, it seems, don't generally produce significant alterations of consciousness.

## What About Women?

Although yohimbine is known primarily as a treatment for male impotence, we were nevertheless surprised that the literature researched for this chapter did not contain *a single reference* to yohimbine's effects in women. The only even remotely relevant statement was found in the *Physicians' Desk Reference*: "Generally, this drug is not proposed for use in females" [PDR, 1994].

The very *absence* of data in this area leaves open the possibility that this substance may offer substantial prosexual benefits to women. (Most prosexual drugs, after all, appear to work for both sexes.) And the few isolated bits of evidence that we *have* managed to gather—from animal research and personal interviews—hint at exciting prospects.

A study published in 1985 reports that "yohimbine induced mounting in...nonreceptive female rats." In other words, this compound stimulated sexual activity in female rats during a stage of their sexual cycle normally characterized by the complete *absence* of such behavior—a noteworthy finding. In a study with female rats in heat, yohimbine was able to counteract the suppression of sexually receptive behavior induced by another compound [Davis, 1977].

> "There have been no studies to date of yohimbine's effects on sexual function in women."
> —Rosen and Ashton
> *Prosexual Drugs...*

Two of the women interviewed for this book have each performed a single experiment with yohimbine. Both report positive results, and neither experienced any negative effects.

The first, a woman in her early forties, used an herbal yohimbe product that produced "a delicious sense of spreading sensation, and a tingling in the pelvic area."

The second woman, who was thirty-four years old, took 16.2 milligrams (3 tablets) of prescription yohimbine and fell asleep shortly thereafter. She had a vivid, powerful erotic dream that resulted in an intense orgasm. This incident is especially impressive because *erotic dreams have always been an extremely rare occurrence for this woman—and never before (at least to her knowledge) has she had an orgasm in her sleep.*

### A different kind of prosexual effect

The following anecdote from the interviews conducted for this book describes what might be called an "indirect route of action" by which this compound can affect women.

A woman in her early thirties expresses tremendous enthusiasm for yohimbine, insisting that its benefits for women are *at least* as great as those experienced by men. She takes so much pleasure in this compound's effects that, when arranging a date with her male partner, she always reminds him repeatedly, "don't forget to bring the yohimbine!"

Of course, it is *his* use of the compound—and the results—that provide her with such delight. This woman clearly obtains prosexual effects from yohimbine even though she never actually ingests it herself.

## Safety Issues

Yohimbine therapy for impotence has been referred to as "a safe treatment" [Reid, 1987]. In one large study of yohimbine's efficacy in treating impotence among elderly patients, "a higher rate of adverse side effects was reported in patients on placebo, as compared to drug treatment" [Rosen, 1993].

The overall safety of yohimbine is illustrated by an incident of overdose reported in a medical journal. A sixty-two year-old man took *200 milligrams* of yohimbine hydrochloride—around *fourty times* the dosage range usually used for therapeutic purposes. "The only adverse effects," according to the summary of the report, "were tachycardia [rapid heartbeat], hypertension, and anxiety of brief duration." The authors conclude that "the limited experience to date suggests a benign course even after massive overdose" [Friesen, 1993].

### Side effects

Yohimbine and yohimbe products can cause anxiety. In fact, yohimbine has been called a "model anxiety-producing agent" [Buffum, 1982]. While this effect usually requires very large doses, one man interviewed for this book experienced this reaction in response to a single dose of a relatively mild herbal tincture.

Other side effects and adverse reactions can include: nausea, vomiting, increased blood pressure, excessive sweating, overstimulation, salivation, elevated heart rate, tremor, irritability, incoordination, dizziness, headache, and skin flushing [PDR, 1994; Grossman, 1993; Hollander, 1992; Yates, 1991].

The typical dose of yohimbine used in impotence therapy has been described as having "little side effect" [Sonda, 1990].

### Contraindications

According to the *Physicians' Desk Reference*, yohimbine should not be used by geriatric patients, pregnant women, children, people with kidney problems, or people with histories of gastric or duodenal ulcer. The *PDR* also cautions against the use of yohimbine in psychiatric patients or in conjunction with antidepressants and other mood-modifying drugs [PDR, 1994].

Researchers investigating yohimbine's effects on blood pressure and norepinephrine activity concluded that "yohimbine should be administered with caution to patients with high blood pressure, especially in individuals...undergoing concurrent treatment with tricyclic antidepressants or other drugs that interfere with neuronal uptake or metabolism of norepinephrine" [Grossman, 1993]. Readers should note that deprenyl, a compound serving as the topic for one of the chapters in this book, interferes with uptake of norepinephrine and is used as an antidepressant. It may therefore be inadvisable to use deprenyl in conjunction with yohimbine, especially for those who have high blood pressure.

Cautions and contraindications applying to yohimbine should also be applied to over-the-counter herbal yohimbe preparations.

## Dosages

Tablets of prescription yohimbine hydrochloride contain 5.4 milligrams each. Dosages used in the treatment of sexual dysfunction range from 16.2 milligrams per day (three tablets) [Jacobsen, 1992] to forty-two milligrams (eight tablets) per day [Susset, 1989].

The quantity of yohimbine hydrochloride present in herbal yohimbe products varies drastically. One analysis of ten brands conducted a few years ago found that the dose per capsule or tablet ranged from 4.5 milligrams to 14.4 milligrams [Griffin, 1991].

Those using yohimbine or yohimbe products occasionally for sex-enhancement purposes will have to determine their own appropriate dosage levels through *cautious* experimentation. Effects of a sufficient dose usually begin within an hour. Some people prefer taking small quantities intermittently beginning several hours or even a day in advance of an anticipated sexual encounter. Others take a single larger dose shortly beforehand. Keep in mind, however, that some of the effects of yohimbe, as mentioned above, can take two to three weeks to kick in.

## Legality and Availability

A wide variety of yohimbe bark extracts are available over-the-counter at health food stores and other outlets for herbal supplements, as well as by mail order. These come in the form of capsules and tinctures.

Yohimbine hydrochloride can be obtained in tablet form by prescription in the United States.

## Physicians and Product Sources

Please note the tearout card at the front of this book where you will find instructions for getting our *Directory of Mail Order Pharmacies* and *Directory of Physicians*. These listings are updated monthly. (Please also read the 'Disclaimer' section at the front of this book.)

# Part II:

# Synthetic Substances

*"I take 5 milligrams of bromocriptine every night before going to bed. Since I started using it, I never fail to awaken with an erection... And my dreams are very explicitly erotic."*

—49 year-old man who had no erectile problems before using bromocriptine

# Bromocriptine

## *Prosexual uses of Bromocriptine:* ────────────

Men:    increased interest/desire; increased erectile capacity; ease of ejaculation & postponing ejaculation; increased subjective enjoyment.

Women:   increased interest/desire; increased frequency of orgasm.

## What is Bromocriptine?

Bromocriptine is nearly miraculous for its multiplicity of beneficial effects. While at present it is used primarily in the treatment of Parkinson's disease, the research performed so far suggests roles for this compound in life extension, cognition enhancement, fat reduction, mood modulation, increasing immunity, sex enhancement, and treating sexual dysfunction.

Perhaps no less should be expected from a member of such an illustrious family. Bromocriptine's diverse chemical cousins include both the notorious psychedelic LSD and hydergine, a treatment for senility and a favorite among users of smart drugs. This noble molecular bloodline can be traced back to humble origins in *ergot*, a species of mold that grows on rye. Several of these semisynthetic ergot derivatives, among them LSD and hydergine, were developed by the famous Swiss chemist Albert Hofmann and marketed by his

## *Actual and Possible Uses of Bromocriptine*

**Treatment of:**
Parkinsonism (alone or in conjunction with L-dopa)
Alzheimer's disease
Pituitary tumors
Hyperprolactinemia
Sex disorders related to hyperprolactinemia and pituitary
    tumors
Sex dysfunction in kidney failure patients undergoing
    hemodialysis
Sex dysfunction due to antipsychotics
Cocaine abuse & withdrawal
Sex disorders related to cocaine abuse
Acromegaly
Certain sleep disorders
Prostate enlargement
Incomplete sexual development
Breast cancer (& prevention)
Breast engorgement in women bottle-feeding their
    newborns
Breast pain associated with the menstrual cycle
Pre-menstrual syndrome
Mild to moderate hypertension
Depression
Diabetes type II
Obesity
Shock & stress
Alcoholism & related sexual dysfunction
Low sperm count in men and infertility in men and women

**And for:**
Fat reduction
Life extension
Immune enhancement
Normalizing levels of dopamine, testosterone, growth
    hormone
Increasing lean muscle mass/fat ratio
Cognition enhancement, particularly in regard to "working
    memory"

**And as:**
An antioxidant
A prosexual drug

employer, Sandoz Laboratories. Bromocriptine, one ergot derivative not associated with Hofmann, has been distributed by Sandoz under the name Parlodel for approximately two decades.

Bromocriptine is a potent dopaminergic, meaning that it is a stimulant (or *agonist*) of the brain's dopamine system. This system plays a crucial role in sexuality (see the chapter entitled "Some Basic Physiology") [Julien, 1988].

Two primary types of receptor sites—molecular docking bays where neurotransmitters temporarily bind to a cell and change its chemical state—have been isolated for dopamine. These have been named "D1" and "D2" and have been identified with two complementary subsystems of the dopamine system featuring different (and sometimes even opposing) functions. For instance, D2 has been associated with cognition and D1 with motor functions. The action of bromocriptine has been found to be highly specific to D2 receptor sites [Block, 1993].

The prosexual effects of bromocriptine are attributed to its dopaminergic properties, its ability to decrease levels of the hormone prolactin, and its capacity to increase concentrations of testosterone when they are low [Stegmayr, 1985; Vircburger, 1985; Winters, 1984].

Bromocriptine is considered relatively safe and non-toxic. (See "Precautions, Side Effects, and Contraindications" below).

## Bromocriptine's Balancing Quality

Perhaps the most remarkable property of bromocriptine is its balancing, normalizing, regulatory, or buffering action on certain hormones. This quality provides an inherent safety mechanism with regard to at least some of its effects. For instance, bromocriptine will raise dopamine levels when they are low, but will bring them down when they are high [Pearson, 1982; Werner, 1978; Besser, 1978].

Presumably, this built-in safety valve would protect some users of bromocriptine from the side effects of extremely high levels of growth hormone or from the manic and paranoid states connected with super-high dopamine concentrations. In fact, none of the research that we have encountered associates the use of this drug by itself with dangerously low or dangerously high levels of any hormones.

## Bromocriptine, Aging, & Sex

Prolactin is a hormone secreted by the pituitary gland. In women, it stimulates breast engorgement and lactation. High levels of prolactin—a condition known as *hyperprolactinemia*—cause sex negative effects in both men and women, particularly impotence in men [Buvat, 1985]. Foremost among the causes of high prolactin levels are aging, kidney failure, and prolactin-secreting *adenomas*, or tumors, of the pituitary gland, known as *prolactinomas* (discussed below) [Konig, 1986].

Normal aging is associated with lower levels of dopamine and increased levels of prolactin. The prolactin increase normally associated with aging may not be sufficient to receive a diagnosis of "hyperprolactinemia" from a doctor but could, nevertheless, cause some lessening of the sexual vigor associated with youth. Bromocriptine may help by reversing this hormonal change.

We have encountered no studies directly investigating bromocriptine's possible function as a life-extender in either human or animal subjects. However, like other compounds (notably deprenyl and L-dopa) whose promise in this capacity has been verified in animals, bromocriptine is a dopamine agonist. Furthermore, bromocriptine combats many of the syndromes associated with aging: decay of the dopamine system, decrease in testosterone, increases in prolactin, and associated loss of immune function (see below). In a development suggestive of astonishing anti-aging potential, bromocriptine has returned menstruation to some postmenopausal women, and has been shown to have this effect in *most* aging female rats [Pearson, 1982].

It is also possible that bromocriptine interferes with a specific form of age-related brain deterioration: the incorporation of sugar into the tissue of a brain region called the hippocampus. This phenomenon did not occur when bromocriptine was present in cultures of hippocampal tissue taken from rats [Block, 1993].

In their authoritative work, *The Neuroendocrine Theory of*

"On my first two sexual occasions after a dry spell of several months, I was unpleasantly surprised by almost total impotence. I'd been with this partner many times before, and nothing like this had ever happened. I could tell she was disappointed, and I was both frustrated and disturbed.

"A few weeks after this I started taking bromocriptine in tiny amounts, starting with one milligram per day and slowly working my way up to 2.5 milligrams per day split into morning and bedtime doses.

"I almost *never* have erotic dreams—maybe one or two a year. But during the first ten days on bromocriptine, I had *three* intense erotic dreams (and, of course, maybe even more that I don't remember). And I started waking up in the morning with a hard-on, which hadn't been happening very often lately.

"After only eleven days on bromocriptine, I spent three sex-filled days and nights with a new partner. She was incredibly sexy, but I can't imagine that the added thrill of being with someone new could explain the unbelievable difference in my potency as compared to my last encounters. In fact, I was far more potent than ever before.

"I was fully erect, or very close to it, for the entire six or seven hours of our first session. (This is no exaggeration—I happened to glance at the bedside clock just before we started and just after we finished.) And when I finally had my orgasm, it was super-powerful. The next day I ejaculated *three times* in *one hour*—without even softening up that much in between. This level of stamina persisted for all three days.

"I was completely amazed and delighted—as was my new lover."

—31-year-old male

*Aging and Degenerative Disease*, doctors Vladimir Dilman and Ward Dean recommend bromocriptine as one of several substances that "should be considered for their effect on aging and diseases of aging" [Dilman, 1992]. Bromocriptine is discussed at several points by researchers Durk Pearson and Sandy Shaw in *Life Extension*, particularly in its capacity as a growth hormone releaser (although Dilman and Dean suggest that its efficacy as such in the middle-aged and older "has yet to be confirmed"). Bromocriptine, at five milligrams per day, is part of the experimental life extension program that Pearson and Shaw use on themselves (but they go to great lengths to make clear that they are *not* recommending this regimen for use by others).

## Bromocriptine, Prolactin, & Sex

In cases of prolactinoma (prolactin-secreting pituitary tumor), there is a rough positive correlation between prolactin levels and tumor size [Katzir, 1990]. It is possible that, at least in men, *most* cases of hyperprolactinemia are caused by such tumors [Schwartz, 1982; Eversmann, 1981]. Other causes include pregnancy and lactation, the use of antipsychotics and prescribed estrogens, cirrhosis of the liver, hypothyroidism, and chronic kidney failure [Konig, 1986]. As mentioned earlier, prolactin levels also naturally increase with aging [Dilman, 1992].

Estimates of the proportion of cases of impotence that are caused by hyperprolactinemia range from as low as 3% to as high as 25% [Buvat, 1985; el-Beheiry, 1988; Pearson, 1982]. In one study of 135 men suffering from impotence, ejaculatory problems, decreased libido, or some combination thereof, 8.1% were diagnosed with hyperprolactinemia [Schwartz, 1982]. The vast disparity among these estimates may be partly due to differences in the concentration of prolactin levels required to constitute a hyperprolactinemic diagnosis.

In addition to impotence and decreased drive, sex-related symptoms of hyperprolactinemia in men may include premature ejaculation, inability to ejaculate, infertility due to low sperm count or loss of sperm motility, low testosterone levels, galactorrhea (lactation, usually during night), gynecomastia (breast enlargement), enlarged prostate, and painful hypersensitivity of the testicles [Pearson, 1982].

Because of the possibility of an underlying prolactinoma—a very treatable condition—it is recommended that you have your prolactin levels checked if you suffer from any of these symptoms. This advice applies especially strongly in the case of male impotence [Foster, 1990].

Impotence can be an early warning sign of a pituitary tumor. Especially if impotence occurs suddenly, have your prolactin levels checked.

It is not necessarily standard procedure for a general practitioner or urologist to assess hormone levels when presented with a case of impotence or other sexual dysfunction. If a hormonal assay is performed, the hormone concentration most likely to be checked, at least in men, is that of testosterone.

However, although this possibility is not well-known, *prolactin levels can be high—and can result in impotence—even when testosterone levels are normal* [Buvat, 1985].

If your prolactin levels are high, have yourself checked radiologically for the presence of a pituitary tumor. If a tumor is found, bromocriptine, which stands a good chance of solving the sexual symptoms, will probably be part of your treatment [Katzir, 1990]. If prolactin levels are high but no tumor is found, a relatively moderate regular dose of bromocriptine is even more likely to normalize your prolactin levels *and* restore sexual capacity rapidly.

In women, hyperprolactinemia manifests as depressed libido, inappropriate lactation, menstrual irregularity or lack of menstruation (amenorrhea), infertility due to anovulation, hirsutism (hairiness), and mild depression.

Headache and decrease of visual field can be added to the list of symptoms when the larger variety of pituitary tumor is present. This kind of prolactinoma occurs more often in men than in women [Koppelman, 1987; Eversmann, 1981; Kirby, 1979; Konig, 1986].

In any case, half or more of those diagnosed with hyperpro-lactinemia suffer deleterious sexual effects [Moussa, 1985;

Eversmann, 1981].

Bromocriptine is considered "the treatment of choice" for pituitary prolactinomas, as well as for infertility and lack of menstruation caused by hyperprolactinemia in women [Bergh, 1978]. It is also effective in the treatment of male infertility related to prolactin imbalance [Okkens, 1992; Ermolenko, 1986; Tsakok, 1985; Ayalon, 1982].

Bromocriptine has repeatedly been shown to be more than 80% effective in normalizing prolactin levels in hyperprolactinemic patients both with and without pituitary tumors. In one study of 11 patients, prolactin concentrations decreased to an average of 1.7% of pre-treatment levels [Sobrinho, 1981; Lamberts, 1991; Katzir, 1990; Buffum, 1982]. Tumor growth is controlled, and tumor shrinkage occurs in more than half of those treated [Ciccarelli, 1993]. In fact, bromocriptine can sometimes serve as a replacement for pituitary surgery [Mbanya, 1993]. In one instance, after a single injection of 50 milligrams of a long-acting, injectable form of bromocriptine, "a very large tumor virtually disappeared" [Kocijancic, 1990].

A reduction in prolactin levels may drastically improve sexual function and libido. In several studies, success in the sexual arena occurred in *all* of those treated who had suffered problems in this area, at least among the men [Ciccarelli, 1993; Katzir, 1990; el-Beheiry, 1988; Werder, 1978; Sobrinho, 1981]. (In the dozens of reports we have studied, data on this issue regarding women are less frequently included, and even when they do appear they are often stated in rather vague terms. A section focusing specifically on bromocriptine's sexual effects in women appears below.)

One study produced overall results so remarkable as to be worth recounting in some detail. In this instance, all results were obtained from only a *single* dose of 50 milligrams of the injectable, long-acting form of bromocriptine mentioned above. Thirteen patients—eight women and five men—were so treated. Five had macroadenomas, the larger form of prolactin-secreting pituitary tumors, and eight had microadenomas, the smaller form. In those with macroadenomas, prolactin levels fell sharply within twelve hours of the injection; in one patient, a "normal" concentration was reached within this time period, as was the case with *seven of the eight* who suffered from microadenomas. Prolactin suppression in all cases persisted for a minimum of twenty-eight days, and tumor size decreased from 20% to 59% in the first twenty-one days following the injection. All three patients who had visual symptoms showed improvement. Within seven to forty-one days, menstruation returned in all six of the women who had suffered amenorrhea. Galactorrhea vanished in all four of the thirteen patients who had exhibited this symptom. In the two men whose tumors were of the smaller variety, libido and potency were restored to "normal" levels. Adverse side effects were considered brief in duration and only "mild to

### Pearson, prolactin, and Parlodel

"At 17, I was diagnosed as having varicose veins in my legs (correct) and in my testicles (incorrect, but understandable). My testicles were painfully sensitive to slight pressure and did indeed feel varicose. I discovered the real problem about a dozen years ago: hyperprolactinemia...In most men, hyperprolactinemia causes loss of libido and potency, but fortunately I was in the minority not so affected. This condition does not usually cause male gynecomastia (breast enlargement), and I exhibited none. It does sometimes cause lactation, and indeed occasional traces of nocturnal lactation could be found on my sheets.

"...I obtained some bromocriptine from a scientific colleague in Europe. I took an initial dose of 600 micrograms and, within two hours, all testicular hypersensitivity had vanished...Several hours later, things were back to their usual state. So long as I take a total of about 3 mg of bromocriptine (divided into four doses) per day, the apparent varicosity and painful hypersensitivity of the testicles, and the nocturnal trace lactation remain absent. The testicular symptoms promptly return whenever I miss a dose, and just as promptly vanish once again when I take it."

—Durk Pearson
*Life Extension: A Practical Scientific Approach*

moderate" in intensity [Montini, 1986].

Somewhat less consistently than its reduction of prolactin, bromocriptine also restores testosterone levels in cases of hyperprolactinemia, although this takes longer than prolactin inhibition, which begins one or two hours after administration [Winters, 1984; Pearson, 1982]. Some improvement in sex function has been reported even among those for whom bromocriptine has lowered prolactin *without* concomitant restoration of testosterone levels. In such cases, synergetic treatment with exogenous testosterone can be used to maximize sexual recovery [Rigaud, 1992; Nagulesparen, 1978].

Bromocriptine also has an excellent record of restoring libido and sexual function in hyperprolactinemic patients undergoing long-term dialysis for kidney failure (or *uremia*). In a study of thirty-eight men and twenty-one women undergoing long-term maintenance hemodialysis for this condition, about half of the patients reported sexual dysfunction. Among these, prolactin levels were found to be significantly higher than among those reporting no such disturbances. Bromocriptine was administered to five of the hyperprolactinemic patients reporting sexual dysfunction; the treatment normalized prolactin levels and improved sexual function in all of these [Weizman, 1983].

Another study found high prolactin levels among precisely half—seventeen out of thirty-four—male uremic patients on long-term hemodialysis. Of these, the seven "most impotent" were given daily doses of bromocriptine. In all of these patients, prolactin concentrations were reduced to normal levels within four weeks, accompanied by an increase in testosterone. The men all reported a concomitant increase in libido and potency [Vircburger, 1985]. Another report claims that daily doses of bromocriptine improved sexual function in six out of seven uremic patients undergoing chronic hemodialysis [Buffum, 1982].

One study of the use of bromocriptine to treat sexual dysfunction in impotent men on hemodialysis is worthy of special attention due to its methodological integrity. This experiment was of the double-blind, placebo controlled crossover variety (see "Our Research Methods" in the Introduction). Here, bromocriptine resulted in the improvement of "libido or the frequency and/or quality of erections" in eleven out of fourteen male subjects. Interestingly, the failure of bromocriptine in the remaining three cases is correlated with low initial testosterone levels, which presumably failed to improve [Muir, 1983]. Another methodologically rigorous study on male hemodialysis patients reports marked improvement of sexual function concomitant with a consistent reduction of prolactin levels [Bommer, 1979].

The balance of evidence strongly indicates that bromocriptine is an effective treatment for sexual problems related to hyperprolactinemia, especially impotence in men.

## Bromocriptine and the Sexual Side Effects of Other Medications

Bromocriptine is sometimes used to treat sexual problems that occur with the use of a class of psychiatric medications known as major tranquilizers, neuroleptics, or antipsychotics [Sullivan, 1990]. Sexual side effects of these compounds in men include alterations in libido, and problems with erection and ejaculation (and, oddly enough, in some cases "priapism," persistent erection in the absence of sexual stimulation). In women, menstrual irregularities, lessening of libido, and inability to orgasm can occur [Sullivan, 1990].

Neuroleptics control psychotic states by inhibiting dopamine activity in the brain, excesses of which in certain brain areas have been linked to schizophrenic states. Decreases in libido and other sexual problems are often attributed to this antidopaminergic effect [Martin-Du Pan, 1978]. And, at least some of these medications stimulate the release of prolactin. Thorazine, for instance, can be expected to result in a 50% or greater increase of prolactin levels within one hour of administration to healthy men and women, although this effect is less dramatic in older people [Dilman, 1992].

The employment of dopamine-stimulating drugs (as well as growth-hormone releasers) among those using neuroleptics for antipsychotic purposes may be problematic, precisely because of the correlation between high dopamine levels and psychosis. Durk Pearson and Sandy Shaw warn that doses of bromocriptine greater than 30 milligrams per day (a very high dose—more than twice the highest recommended therapeutic dose for Parkinson's disease) can aggravate schizophrenic symptoms [Pearson, 1982].

## Bromocriptine and L-dopa in the Treatment of Parkinsonism

One of bromocriptine's two approved uses in the United States is the treatment of Parkinson's disease, an age-related syndrome believed to be caused by degradation of the dopamine system. In this capacity bromocriptine is used as an adjunct to L-dopa, the standard treatment for Parkinsonism. Its addition to L-dopa sometimes results in a more effective therapy [Grimes, 1983]. One study records a 20% to 37% improvement in symptoms among those in whom L-dopa treatment alone had proven inadequate [Toyokura, 1985].

L-dopa is an amino acid that functions as a dopamine *precursor*, meaning that the body converts this substance into dopamine itself. The high doses of L-dopa administered to Parkinson's patients are sometimes associated with adverse side effects that some sufferers find difficult to tolerate. Bromocriptine is associated with fewer side effects [Pearson, 1982]. Furthermore, L-dopa may actually accelerate the damage to the dopamine system whose symptoms it is used to treat [Pearson, 1982]. The enzyme monoamine oxidase (MAO), found in the brain as well as the digestive tract, is responsible for the breakdown of dopamine into oxidative "free radicals" that cause cell damage. MAO activity increases with age, thus contributing to both the age-related decrease of dopamine levels *and* to greater levels of the dopamine metabolites thought to play a role in Parkinsonism. Not only does L-dopa increase dopamine levels—and therefore the levels of free radicals created from dopamine by MAO—but *itself* oxidizes into free radicals.

Bromocriptine is not oxidized in this fashion. Because of its structural similarity to hydergine, a known *antioxidant* (an agent that interferes with the activity of free radicals), some have even speculated that bromocriptine may also function as an antioxidant [Block, 1993; Pearson, 1982]. Such action would afford bromocriptine even greater value in Parkinsonism.

In order to curb the unwanted effects of L-dopa in treating Parkinsonism, including free-radical damage, bromocriptine can be used to replace approximately half of the L-dopa usually ingested. The resulting treatment usually seems to be as effective as L-dopa alone, and is often accompanied by decreased side-effects and less long-term degeneration—and in some cases, the apparent reversal of such degeneration [Pearson, 1982]. These results support the possibility of antioxidative action.

The use of dopaminergic drugs in Parkinson's has been associated with restoration of libido and sexual function, and in some cases even with outbursts of "hypersexuality." (More discussion of this subject is available in the section on L-dopa.) One journalist reported a rumor that a research effort using bromocriptine in conjunction with L-dopa for Parkinsonism "was cancelled when many of the elderly people in the study began having sex, and two women over 60 years of age got pregnant." This last prospect—pregnancy—seems plausible in light of the fact that bromocriptine (as mentioned above) has been known to restore menstruation to some postmenopausal women, and regularly does so in aging female rats [Huang, 1976].

## Immunity

Bromocriptine has very recently been employed with some success in the treatment of breast cancer [Block, 1993]. Furthermore, it has totally prevented the induction of breast cancer in rats by quantities of the carcinogen DMBA so large that it would usually induce cancer in every animal. This result points toward a possible *preventive* role for bromocriptine in breast cancer. This possibility is strengthened by suggestions that the compound could be used to prevent recurrence (and presumably initiation) of pituitary tumors and by the beneficial effects demonstrated by growth hormone releasers in animals given cancer [Werder, 1978; Pearson, 1982].

Furthermore, very recently the presence of D2 receptor sites has been tentatively detected on the surfaces of T-cells—cellular agents of immunity that play an important role in fighting cancer—as well as on another type of immune cell. These findings suggest the possibility of immune stimulation by D2 agonists such as bromocriptine [Block, 1993].

## Cognition Enhancement

As might be expected from its structural similarity to hydergine and its functional relationship to deprenyl, bromocriptine shows promise as a smart drug. Bromocriptine's action is specific to the D2 dopamine subsystem, a significant network within our cognitive apparatus.

In methodologically rigorous research, bromocriptine has demonstrated marked enhancement of a cognitive process known as *visuospatial working memory*. The term "visuospatial" refers to the ability to respond to the locations of objects in space through visual perception. "Working memory" refers to a dimension of recall lying between short-term and long-term memory, where information is temporarily stored for quick access and use before it is forgotten or filed in long-term storage.

A double blind, placebo-controlled crossover study tested the ability of healthy women to remember accurately the location of a point of light flashed on a circular screen, both immediately after the flash occurred and eight seconds later. Although bromocriptine showed no effect on immediate response, it improved accuracy after the eight-second delay by 44% over the women's "baseline" levels as determined on placebo [Block, 1993].

One recent study with bromocriptine showed improvement of memory in mice within a certain dosage range, whereas higher dosages had the opposite effect. And, another experiment found bromocriptine helpful in a case of cognitive impairment due to brain damage [Block, 1993].

## Reduction of Body Fat

Bromocriptine may also assist in the loss of body fat by reducing prolactin levels [Cincotta, 1989]. Prolactin stimulates fat synthesis. Such an effect is desirable during pregnancy and breast feeding, times when prolactin is released in large amounts and stimulates milk production. In other cases, reducing prolactin levels (which will not cause fat to be burned, but will nevertheless inhibit synthesis of new fat) could be valuable.

## Other Uses & Effects

Other ways that bromocriptine has been used, or might possibly be used, are myriad:

*High blood pressure:* It is effective in treating mild to moderate hypertension (high blood pressure). This property is a result of vasodilation and may also be linked to reduction of prolactin, high levels of which are associated with hypertension [Dilman, 1992]. (Vasodilation, when it increases blood flow to the genitalia, can also enhance sexual function, particularly male erection.)

*Cocaine withdrawal:* Bromocriptine is among the top four drugs used to treat withdrawal from cocaine and to support abstinence thereafter [Block, 1993]. Cocaine triggers the release of stored dopamine (which is responsible for the cocaine "high"). Use of cocaine can result in depletion of dopamine, which can lead to craving for the drug (or, more specifically, the dopamine activity that it stimulates). In fact, many addicts may have been attracted to cocaine because of an initial dopamine deficiency, a condition which they self-medicate with a drug that provides short-term relief but in the long term only exacerbates the original imbalance. Bromocriptine helps to restore healthy dopamine activity and thereby reduces cravings. It has also been used to treat sexual dysfunction related to cocaine abuse [Cocores, 1986].

*Depression:* Bromocriptine may also function as an antidepressant. In recent experiments, rats that had been exposed to excessive stress exhibited a syndrome paralleling human depression. Bromocriptine was used successfully to reverse this condition [Block, 1993]. Another study found bromocriptine effective for treating the mild depression that sometimes occurs in women with hyperprolactinemia [Koppelman, 1987]. These results are not surprising, since bromocriptine is known to stimulate dopamine activity, low levels of which sometimes play a role in depression.

*Acromegaly:* Bromocriptine has been hailed as a "major advance" in treating acromegaly (or *giantism*), a condition characterized by over activity of the pituitary and excessive levels of growth hormone. Symptoms of acromegaly include sweating, oversized hands and feet, lethargy, low libido, and swelling of soft tissues resulting in distorted facial appearance. Bromocriptine is used in the treatment of this syndrome to reduce growth hormone levels [Besser, 1978; Van Loon, 1977; Staub, 1983].

Bromocriptine has also demonstrated value in treating certain sleep disorders, some cases of incomplete sexual development or delayed puberty, and breast engorgement in women who are bottle-feeding their babies. Its use has been explored in the treatment of diabetes, pre-menstrual syndrome, withdrawal from alcohol, treating prostate enlargement, and the treatment of Alzheimer's [Dean, 1992; Koenig, 1977; Block, 1993; Pearson, 1982].

Animal studies suggest yet more possible roles for this amazingly diverse medicine. These include treating alcohol addiction and related sexual dysfunction, reversing effects of stress, and managing states of physiological shock [Andronova, 1987; Kaliszuk, 1989; Block, 1993].

## Other Prosexual Possibilities

So far the discussion of bromocriptine's sexual effects have focussed on the treatment of sexual dysfunction related to hyperprolactinemia. Is bromocriptine valuable where sexual problems have other origins? Can it be used in a prosexual capacity by those have no sexual deficits *per se*, but who seek to enhance and enrich an already "functional" sex life? The jury is still out on these questions, but there are some encouraging data.

Two studies on male impotence in the absence of hormonal imbalance reported that bromocriptine was *not* helpful [Buffum, 1982]. In contrast, a methodologically rigorous investigation of the efficacy of dopaminergic agents in cases of male impotence tied to diabetes offers a more hopeful perspective. While hormonal assays of the men in this study showed no significant differences from a healthy control group, bromocriptine was reported to be 20% more effective than placebo [Pierini, 1981].

Since it is a stimulant of the dopamine system and a booster of testosterone, there are a number of good reasons to suspect that bromocriptine would be prosexual among those who consider themselves sexually "normal and healthy"—as did the forty-nine year-old man whose report opens this chapter. Evidence in support of such a possibility includes the fact that injections of bromocriptine were used to induce erection in male animals [Block, 1993].

Gerontologist and smart drug authority Ward Dean, MD, considers small doses of bromocriptine sufficiently safe to use as an experimental prosexual drug.

## ... And What About Women?

Since the balance of hard data regarding bromocriptine's sexual effects—both in this discussion so far as well as in the sources from which it has been drawn—has focused on men, it seems worthwhile to sift out and pull together some of the scattered information relevant to women and offer it special treatment.

The same factors just mentioned regarding bromocriptine's general prosexual utility—effects on the dopamine system and levels of prolactin and testosterone—support the notion of bromocriptine as a sex-enhancer for women. The data that *do* exist in this area are quite positive:

→   "Improved libido" was reported in a fertility-oriented study of forty-two women. The women were all hyperprolactinemic and were given bromocriptine for a prolonged period of time [Bergh, 1978]. (Among women in whom ovulation is reinstated by bromocriptine, it seems logical to expect return of the libido often associated with that portion of the menstrual cycle.)

→   In contrast, another study found no overall differences in libido when bromocriptine was compared to placebo. The study was a double-blind crossover study of only six hyperprolactinemic and six "normal" women. However, one of the hyperprolactinemic women had orgasms *only* during the portion of the experiment when she was administered bromocriptine [Koppelman, 1987]. In such a small sample, this woman alone accounts for approximately 16% of the hyperprolactinemic cases and 8% of the total.

→    Two women in a study of bromocriptine's efficacy in shrinking macroprolactinomas reported their first orgasms in many years [Sobrinho, 1981].

→    Further suggestive evidence comes from the realm of animal studies. Low doses of other dopaminergic drugs have been found to increase the sexual receptivity of female rats, and low doses of bromocriptine itself enhanced "proceptivity" (sex-initiating behavior) among female rhesus monkeys [Everitt, 1978]. Given that these animals were in healthy condition to begin with, such results bode well for bromocriptine's potential as a prosexual substance in normal, healthy human females.

## Safety Issues

The side effects most commonly associated with bromocriptine do not result from toxicity on the part of the drug itself, but instead are linked to stimulation of the dopamine system (and are therefore common to other dopaminergic drugs) [Pearson, 1982; Julien, 1988]. The most common are nausea and vomiting. Dizziness, lowered blood pressure, increased blood pressure, headache, and manic-like over stimulation (sometimes called "behavioral arousal") are other possible side effects [PDR, 1984].

Other more serious complications and reactions have been reported, but are very rare [Moussa, 1985; Landolt, 1985; Blin, 1991]. One source estimates that such incidents take place in a fraction of one percent of all users [Block, 1993]. Particular attention has recently been paid to some cases of hypertension, seizure, and stroke that have occurred in women who were taking bromocriptine to prevent lactation after pregnancy—although the relationship of these incidents to the use of bromocriptine is not clear [PDR, 1994]. More information on these cases can be found in *The Physicians' Desk Reference.*

Most studies seem to agree that side effects are usually mild or moderate, easily tolerated, tend to disappear after the first few days of therapy or sooner, and occur in a minority of those treated (25%, according to one report). It seems possible that a slightly higher incidence of side effects occurs among those undergoing dialysis. One extensive review of the literature with an eye towards long-term safety offered a very positive overall evaluation [Weil, 1986].

To further put matters in perspective: in a study of dialysis patients from which seven of twenty-five men were withdrawn due to side effects of bromocriptine, another man was removed apparently because he poorly tolerated side effects of a *placebo* [Muir, 1983].

In most studies, daily doses of bromocriptine's oral form run in the five to ten milligram range or even lower [Lamberts, 1991; Vircburger, 1985; Bommer, 1979; Buffum 1982]. The safety of such dosage levels is confirmed by cases in which daily dosages have run as high as 60 [Wass, 1977] and even 170 milligrams [Weil, 1986] without, apparently, untoward effect. Bromocriptine's long-acting injectable form has been used at levels as high as 250 milligrams, again without special difficulty [Ciccarelli, 1993].

The side effects of bromocriptine can be modulated—and sometimes completely avoided—by cutting back the dosage or by slowly increasing it from the beginning of use [Pearson, 1982; Besser, 1978].

In response to incidents in which bromocriptine has restored menstrual cycling to postmenopausal women, Pearson and Shaw warn that bromocriptine's use among such individuals should be accompanied by birth control, citing the higher rates of birth defects associated with children born to women late in life [Pearson, 1982].

The only specific contraindications for bromocriptine are: "Uncontrolled hypertension, toxemia of pregnancy, [and] sensitivity to any ergot alkaloids" [PDR 1994]. However, it is possible that, because of its dopaminergic effect, extra caution should be exercised where manic or psychotic conditions or predispositions are present.

## Dosage & Timing

In therapy for hyperprolactinemia, the daily dose of bromocriptine's oral form is usually divided into two or three portions. Similarly, Pearson and Shaw recommended breaking the dosage into two to four daily portions when using bromocriptine for other purposes [Pearson, 1982].

Bromocriptine has been used for prosexual and life extension purposes by many healthy individuals in doses of 1.25 to 5 milligrams daily [Pearson, 1982, Block, 1993].

## Availability and Legal Status

Bromocriptine is available by prescription under the name Parlodel in the United States, where its use is approved for Parkinsonism and syndromes related to hyperprolactinemia. There are no legal barriers for a physician to prescribe it for other uses. Bromocriptine is also available from several overseas mail order pharmacies without a prescription. (Please note, however, that we still recommend that you work with your personal physician.)

## Physicians and Product Sources

Please note the tearout card at the front of this book where you will find instructions for getting our *Directory of Mail Order Pharmacies* and *Directory of Physicians*. These listings are updated monthly. (Please also read the 'Disclaimer' section at the front of this book.)

*"For me, deprenyl is a fantastic boon to sex from a number of angles. First of all, it definitely revs up my sex drive. Plus, the smart drug aspect of it seems to open up the doors of communication—especially if the person I'm with has also taken it. It seems to stimulate, prolong, and deepen conversation, making it sharper, livelier, and somehow sexier. And deprenyl does something to the way my skin feels and the sense of touch that is very sensual and exciting."*

—thirty-year-old man

# Deprenyl

## *Prosexual uses of deprenyl:* ————————————

Women:   increased libido; enhanced subjective experience of sex.

Men:   increased libido; more frequent sexual interest; enhanced subjective experience of sex.

## What Is Deprenyl?

Deprenyl is the most impressive and well-documented life-extending substance known. For this and many other reasons, it will no doubt go down in history along with other molecular "movers and shakers" like Prozac and piracetam as one of the top ten most significant pharmacological discoveries of the late Twentieth century. In the year 1992 alone, over 100 scientific papers dealing with deprenyl were published worldwide [Dean, 1993].

Extensive research on Deprenyl began in the 1950s. This remarkable compound was developed by Dr. Joseph Knoll, a Hungarian who has been called "the father of deprenyl" [Block, 1993]. Knoll, whose research focussed on the clinical uses of amphetamine-like compounds and other stimulants, was originally interested in deprenyl's potential as a treatment for hypertension [Dean, 1993]. Although it did not fulfill its promise in this area, it has proven remarkable in the treatment of Parkinson's disease (for which it has been used by millions), depression, and, most recently, Alzheimer's disease.

The chemical name for deprenyl is *selegiline hydrochloride*, and it is often simply called "selegiline." The molecular structure of deprenyl has been called "a slight, but exceptionally lucky chemical modification" of phenethylamine, or PEA. The latter is a compound "found widely throughout nature, both in plants and animals." While

a rather questionable mythology has evolved around PEA as the "love chemical" present in high concentrations in chocolate, according to psychopharmacologist Alexander T. Shulgin "the jury is still out" as to the nature of its actual role in human physiology and consciousness.

Both the PEA and deprenyl molecules in turn bear close structural relationships with the following compounds: amphetamine; the neurotransmitters norepinephrine and dopamine; phenylalanine, tyrosine, and L-dopa, amino acids used by the body to make these neurotransmitters; and tyramine, a chemical that occurs in some foods and is also one of PEA's metabolic end-products. (Tyramine appears again in the discussion of MAO inhibition that follows). PEA's structure is considered the chemical basis of all of these compounds, which are therefore grouped together as phenethylamines. This name refers to a vast panorama of PEA-based substances which, taken together, play large roles both in natural human biochemistry and in synthetic pharmacology.

## Deprenyl's Special Effects

While deprenyl's chemical structure closely resembles that of many other substances, its activity is unique. As the literature on this chemical repeatedly emphasizes, deprenyl exhibits a "remarkable pharmacological spectrum" of effects [Knoll, 1992].

Perhaps the most astonishing aspect of this compound's action is the manner in which seemingly independent effects converge with precision to serve a particular end result—deprenyl's potent anti-aging property. Deprenyl's various modes of action work together with uncanny synchrony to preserve, protect, and enhance the dopamine system in a small area of the brain known as the *substantia nigra*. This region features the highest concentration of dopamine found anywhere in the brain. Furthermore, the dopamine neurons in this location age more quickly than any other group of brain cells.

> "Deprenyl has a positive effect on my memory and on my ability to verbalize... [and] a very positive effect on my libido."
> —35-year-old man

In fact, Parkinson's disease has come to be understood as a result of the "premature rapid aging" of the substantia nigra [Knoll, 1992]. And it is now becoming clear that the decay of the dopamine system in this area is also central to normal aging.

Quite understandably, it may be difficult for people without backgrounds in pharmacology and the biology of aging to understand what is so special about deprenyl's effects. A metaphor may be in order.

### Deprenyl as spider-man

Imagine the dopamine system of the substantia nigra as a large dam that has sprouted a number of conveniently finger-sized leaks, each several feet apart. These leaks represent the different aspects of this system's aging process.

Suppose that, in order to prevent a flood before the repair crew shows up, we decided to collect some volunteers to go to this dam and plug the leaks with their fingers. Because the leaks in the dam are so many and so far apart, we would normally expect to need several brave volunteers (therapeutic compounds) with rather strong fingers (pharmacological effects) to do the job (slowing down the "leakage" or the aging of the substantia nigra's dopamine system).

Much to our surprise, however, we are approached by a spider-like person (deprenyl) with several long arms of incredible reach (divergent pharmacological effects). He demonstrates his ability to do the job largely on his own.

Suppose further that the area in which the dam has been built (the brain) is part of a national park or preserve that must be kept in pristine condition. We therefore want our spider-man to perform his task without feeding the bears, leaving any litter, picking any flowers, or otherwise disturbing the grounds (in other words, without creating side effects in other parts or systems of the brain). To our utter astonishment, our extraordinary volunteer completes his assignment without leaving so much as a footprint.

Many aspects of deprenyl's action on the dopamine system of the substantia nigra take place with just this kind of precision. Furthermore, as the following material explains, deprenyl features all of several unusual modes of action that are required to bypass a severe toxic reaction (the "cheese effect") common to one of the classes of compounds to which deprenyl belongs.

Here deprenyl presents itself in sharp contrast to the many other drugs which have a broad range of effects on systems of the body other than the one being specifically targeted for therapy. Pharmacologists informally refer to the kind of precision of effect exhibited by deprenyl with the word "clean," as in "a very *clean* compound." (Similarly, substances which feature substantial irrelevant or undesirable secondary effects are sometimes called "dirty.")

The nature of deprenyl's multi-pronged attack on the aging of the substantia nigra's dopamine system makes it seem almost as if this compound were *custom designed* for life-extension purposes. Or, turning this idea on its head, we could say that the human body seems as if it were designed to need deprenyl after a certain age.

These images and metaphors are, of course, less than precise, and they exaggerate the case to a significant degree. We hope, however, that they convey to some extent why deprenyl's effects are worthy of the rather lengthy technical explanations given below. The material that follows, in fact, is probably the most technical passage in this book. Those readers who feel that they have by now gotten the gist of deprenyl's pharmacology, but are not interested in the details, may wish to skip forward to the section entitled "Deprenyl's Subjective Effects."

This rest of this section will concentrate on the following aspects of deprenyl's action: 1) inhibition of the action of a brain enzyme called monamine oxidase B (MAO B); 2) blocking the uptake or absorption into brain cells of a class of neurotransmitters called "catecholamines" as well as related compounds; 3) enhancing the functions by which the substantia nigra protects itself from the damaging effects of free radicals and other toxic substances; and 4) improving the overall functioning of the dopamine system within this area of the brain. All of these functions serve the maintenance and protection of the substantia nigra's dopamine system in different ways. (Remember also that enhancement of dopamine activity has a prosexual effect in most people.)

### But first, a lesson in brain anatomy

Some of the dopamine-using neurons of the substantia nigra extend into a nearby part of the brain known as the striatum. These cells are therefore sometimes referred to as "striatal" or "nigrostriatal" neurons. One of the two major components of the striatum is called the "caudate nucleus." It is shaped something like a curved tail with a bulb at one end. This part of the brain, which is penetrated by the fibers of dopamine neurons originating in the substantia nigra, plays an important role in the discussion of Parkinson's disease in this chapter.

Because these brain regions share dopamine cells, those actions of deprenyl described in the following discussion as preserving or enhancing dopamine function in striatal and nigrostriatal areas can be understood as affecting the substantia nigra's dopamine function in more or less the same manner.

### Inhibition of MAO B

Monamine oxidase (MAO) is an enzyme present both in the digestive tract and in the brain. In the digestive tract, it initiates the metabolic breakdown of various chemicals from foods into forms that can be either assimilated or eliminated by the body.

In the brain, MAO binds to several different neurotransmitters (among them serotonin, norepinephrine, and dopamine) and begins the process of breaking them down into smaller chemical units for eventual elimination from the body.

By way of this neurotransmitter-metabolizing function, MAO plays a significant role in regulating cerebral neurotransmitter levels. Indirectly, therefore, it also plays a part in regulating all of the mental, endocrine, and metabolic functions these brain chemicals affect.

Excessively high levels of MAO will result in significantly decreased concentrations of the neurotransmitters upon which it acts. In the case of dopamine, high levels of MAO might therefore be expected to result in depressed mood and decreased motivation, motor control, cognitive acuity, and sex drive (in other words, a decrease in dopamine-related functions). And, indeed, aging—a process characterized by increasing MAO activity—is all too often accompanied by the symptoms just described.

*MAO inhibitors.* Drugs called "MAO Inhibitors" (MAOIs) block the action of MAO, thereby generating higher levels of those neurotransmitters whose metabolization is initiated by this enzyme. The first substances to achieve widespread clinical use as antidepressants were MAO inhibitors. They were initially derived from a drug being tested as a treatment for tuberculosis. The impetus to investigate possible antidepressive action came from the observation that a ward full of tuberculosis patients classified as "terminally ill" exhibited unusually high spirits while this drug was being tested on them. In fact, their spirits were *so* high that they were regularly seen dancing in the hospital hallways.

*Enter the "cheese effect."* In spite of their excellent track record for alleviating depression, MAOIs were soon replaced as the antidepressants-of-choice by the well-known "tricyclic" antidepressants. The MAOIs fell into relative disfavor because some patients using these drugs experienced mysterious "acute hypertensive crises"—painful and potentially dangerous attacks of high blood pressure. These episodes were traced to a cross-reaction between MAOIs and tyramine, a compound present in the body and various foods. Tyramine occurs in especially high concentrations in aged cheeses. This syndrome has thus become known widely as the *cheese effect.*

Those who use normal doses of deprenyl do not need to worry about the cheese effect. In fact, deprenyl is the only widely used pharmaceutical MAO inhibitor that does not present this problem. (This safety factor allows deprenyl to be administered to Parkinson's patients in conjunction with L-dopa, which would also pose the risk of hypertensive crisis if taken with most MAO inhibitors.) However, some further exploration of the cheese effect will be valuable for understanding both MAO inhibition in general *and* the singular character of deprenyl's pharmacological action.

MAO breaks down tyramine and is thus responsible for keeping a lid on levels of this compound within the body. This function is especially important in protecting the nervous system from toxically high tyramine concentrations.

Most MAO inhibitors interfere with MAO's tyramine-regulating action. Therefore, if such an MAO inhibitor is being used, an excess of tyramine can occur in the nervous system when a high level of this compound is absorbed into the body from a tyramine-rich food.

Tyramine enters certain types of neurons through an absorption process known as *uptake.* Once inside the nerve cell, it displaces stimulatory neurotransmitters called *catecholamines* from *storage granules* where these chemicals are stored in an essentially dormant state. The catecholamines are then released from the neurons into the synapses—the spaces between brain cells—where they perform their stimulatory function.

The catecholamine-releasing action of tyramine, PEA, amphetamines, and other siblings of PEA might be viewed as a process similar to passengers entering and exiting a crowded elevator. As a load of new passengers (tyramine molecules) enter the elevator (a catecholamine storage site inside a brain cell), old passengers (catecholamines) must flood out into the hallway (the synapse) in order to make room for the new passengers.

In the cheese effect, too much tyramine triggers excessive catecholamine release. The resulting sudden surge of catecholamine activity in turn initiates a dangerous increase in blood pressure. (This syndrome is an amplified version of the same kind of blood pressure increase that occurs with amphetamines, which trigger catecholamine release through a route of action similar to that of tyramine.) In worst-case scenarios, the cheese effect can result in fatal brain hemorrhage. Thus, patients taking MAO inhibitors have died from eating a serving of macaroni and cheese [Pearson, 1988].

*MAO A and MAO B.* Knoll's research into deprenyl eventually led to the discovery that there are actually *two* forms of MAO [Knoll, 1992]. One is MAO A, which occurs primarily in the digestive system. The other is MAO B, which occurs primarily in the "glial cells" of the brain. Glial cells have been described as "small brain cells which surround and metabolically support the neurons which conduct the electrical signals throughout the brain" [Dean, 1993].

MAO B is responsible for the breakdown of cerebral dopamine. MAO B activity, and the population of glial cells containing this enzyme, both increase with aging [Dean, 1993]. These factors contribute to the age-associated decrease of dopamine levels and dopamine activity in the brain.

Except at very high doses, deprenyl selectively inhibits MAO B, leaving MAO A untouched. In fact, deprenyl was the first selective MAO B inhibitor described in scientific literature, and remains the only such compound in widespread clinical use [Knoll, 1992].

*Pass the cheese, please.* As mentioned earlier, deprenyl poses no danger of the dreaded "cheese effect" at the dosage levels used for therapeutic, life extension, and prosexual purposes. Part of the reason for deprenyl's special safety factor in this regard is its exclusive inhibition of MAO B. Selective MAO B inhibition does not interfere with the process whereby MAO A in the digestive tract breaks down tyramine from foods. This function of MAO A helps to limit the quantity of dietary tyramine that can eventually cross the blood-brain barrier.

While selective MAO B inhibition is a necessary condition for deprenyl's freedom from the cheese effect, it is not—contrary to much of the popular literature on deprenyl—sufficient in and of itself to guarantee such safety. This is why most of the selective MAO B inhibitors that have been developed since deprenyl still present the potential for hypertensive crisis. At least one additional property—one almost unique among MAO inhibitors—is required. This property will be discussed shortly in the subsection on deprenyl's uptake-blocking effects.

*MAO B inhibition and the substantia nigra.* Deprenyl's selective MAO B inhibition helps to maintain levels of dopamine and dopamine activity throughout the brain, counteracting the dopamine loss usually caused by age-related increases of MAO B activity and growth in glial cell population. MAO B inhibition is of particular value in the substantia nigra area, where, as mentioned earlier, dopamine loss occurs especially rapidly and can have severe consequences (such as contributing to the development of Parkinson's disease).

*The China White Syndrome.* It has been speculated that deprenyl's MAO B inhibition could perform another function vital for protecting the substantia nigra. Young people exposed to a compound known as MPTP (present in some batches of synthetic heroin, or "China White") have rapidly developed full-scale Parkinson's symptoms. This observation has given rise to a theory that Parkinson's may be caused by an MPTP-like toxin.

MAO B converts MPTP into a free radical called $MPP^+$, which specifically damages nigrostriatal dopamine-using neurons. Animal studies have shown that deprenyl—probably by inhibiting MAO B's conversion of MPTP into $MPP^+$—protects the striatum from MPTP toxicity. If the origin of Parkinson's is, in fact, an unknown MPTP-type chemical, it seems reasonably likely that deprenyl would protect the striatal dopamine system from the toxic effects of this "mystery compound" as well [Knoll, 1992; Pearson, 1988].

### Blocking uptake of catecholamines

Both norepinephrine and dopamine are catecholamines—*excitatory* neurotransmitters that Joseph Knoll has described as "the optimum fuel for the engine of the brain" [Knoll, 1992]. As discussed elsewhere in this book, these neurotransmitters are also fuel for sexuality. (Knoll conversely described the brain networks involving serotonin—an *inhibitory* neurotransmitter credited with a dampening effect on libido—as the brain's "brake" system).

Deprenyl blocks the re-uptake—or absorption into brain cells—of norepinephrine and dopamine. (In this function deprenyl stands virtually alone among MAO inhibitors, but resembles "tricyclic" and other antidepressants.) The net effect of this uptake-blocking action is an increase in the levels of these chemicals active in the synapse where neurotransmission occurs.

Deprenyl also blocks the uptake of tyramine, which is similar in structure to norepinephrine and dopamine. As a result, tyramine cannot displace catecholamines from their storage sites inside brain cells. The catecholamine release responsible for the cheese effect's dangerous surge of blood pressure is therefore also prevented.

In terms of the passengers-and-elevator image used earlier to describe tyramine's catecholamine-releasing property, deprenyl acts like a security guard blocking the entrance to the hallway where the elevator is located. Thus, the would-be new elevator passengers (tyramine molecules) don't even get a chance to displace the old passengers (catecholamine molecules) from the elevator (catechol-amine storage site inside a brain cell).

This uptake-blocking action is the second condition (along with selective inhibition of MAO B) necessary for deprenyl's freedom from the cheese effect [Knoll, 1992].

A further uptake-blocking property of deprenyl may be of importance—once again, in protecting the crucial dopamine system of the substantia nigra. Deprenyl blocks the uptake into dopamine active neurons of a compound called 6-OHDA. After uptake, this dopamine metabolite autoxidates (automatically oxidizes) into toxic free radicals that damage the dopamine neurons into which it has been absorbed. 6-OHDA has been used in experiments to simulate

"For me, deprenyl functions amazingly well as a generalized tonic, an overall balancing agent of special value when I'm feeling vaguely out of whack. I don't use deprenyl regularly, but will occasionally take five or ten milligrams in the course of a day when I feel that my stamina, creativity, mental lucidity—or even immunity—could use a special boost.

"Sometimes I still feel foggy and sluggish even though I've had plenty of rest. On those days, a tickle of deprenyl generally puts me right on-line in short order. Oddly enough, however, when I'm tired but too stressed or wired to sleep, a few milligrams of deprenyl will often allow me to drop off quickly into a deep and restful sleep—even though it's generally taken as an energizer or stimulant.

"If I'm slowed down by a cold or hay fever, deprenyl will generally help me feel better. In fact, I've used deprenyl the way many people use the traditional herbal immune-stimulant *echinacea*. Sometimes, if I take deprenyl when I'm beginning to feel the vague but unmistakable signs of incipient cold or flu, I'll take deprenyl—and the infection that seems to be on the way doesn't ever fully kick in.

"In sum, this drug— which feels more like a *nutrient* to me—acts consistently as a general lubricant for my entire system. It seems able to grease the gears and facilitate almost *any* psychophysical process that needs to happen. For instance, there have even been at least a few occasions when mild muscle soreness or joint pain that had been bothering me for days has almost completely dissolved—without coming back later—an hour or so after taking deprenyl.

"I certainly wouldn't expect deprenyl to be as versatile for everyone as it seems to be for me. The broad utility that this compound seems to demonstrate in my individual case probably reflects a highly personal biochemical imbalance or deficiency to which I'm prone. But for me, deprenyl sometimes feels just like mother's milk for my brain."

—Twenty-nine year-old male

Parkinson's disease in monkeys and rats [Knoll, 1986].

6-OHDA appears in particularly high concentrations in the substantia nigra because of the uniquely high dopamine content and activity in this region. It is therefore likely that 6-OHDA plays a role in the nigrostriatal dopamine-system damage characteristic of aging and Parkinson's. By blocking 6-OHDA uptake, deprenyl protects the striatum from such damage [Knoll, 1992].

### Protecting against brain cell damage

There is yet another means by which deprenyl protects the nigrostriatal dopamine system from damage caused by 6-OHDA and other toxic compounds.

Dopa and dopamine are each metabolized into a number of toxic by-products (in addition to 6-OHDA) that damage dopamine neurons. (These by-products fall into two categories: oxidative free radicals and "quinones.") High dopa and dopamine levels— resulting in high levels of their toxic metabolites—may in fact largely explain the unusually rapid aging of the striatal dopamine system. As Joseph Knoll has put it:

> "...dopamine itself might play a main role in the age-related changes of the nigrostriatal dopaminergic neurons...the complex autoxidation of the high amounts of dopamine in the striatum, continuously generating substantial quantities of toxic free radicals and highly reactive quinones, creates a permanent danger for the nigrostriatal dopaminergic neurons, which have to mobilize their natural defensive measures to protect themselves from the deleterious effect of the toxic by-products of dopamine metabolism" [Knoll, 1992].

The "natural defensive measures" mentioned here by Knoll consist of the actions of two enzymes. The first is superoxide dismutase (SOD), a "free radical scavenger" that rounds up and neutralizes the offending molecules like a cerebral vigilante squad. The second enzyme, which performs a similar protective function, is catalase.

Long-term administration of deprenyl has been clearly demonstrated to enhance the activity of *both* SOD *and* catalase in animals. These effects, which kick in after a few weeks of continuous low-dose administration, are *highly specific* to the striatal area in which the protective functions of these enzymes are especially important: they *have not been found to occur in other brain regions.* In this case, deprenyl's marksman-like aim at the bull's-eye of the striatal dopamine system proves most extraordinary.

### Yet more enhancement of dopamine activity

The effects described so far do not exhaust the means by which deprenyl so uncannily zeroes in on the aging of the substantia nigra's dopamine system. In studies with rats, long-term (weeks or months) administration of deprenyl has been conclusively shown to facilitate the overall functioning of the nigrostriatal dopamine system in at least three more ways.

First, deprenyl increases the "firing rate" of striatal dopamine neurons, meaning it causes these cells to emit electrochemical pulses more frequently. Second, deprenyl increases the rate at which these neurons process dopamine (known technically as "efflux" or "turnover rate"). Third, deprenyl increases the release of dopamine from these neurons.

These effects are highly specific to dopamine neurons; similar effects have been sought, but not found, in the nigrostriatal norepinephrine and serotonin systems. Furthermore, Knoll has shown that these effects occur *entirely independently* of deprenyl's MAO inhibition and dopamine-uptake blocking actions. The relevant mechanism remains unknown.

### Other aspects of deprenyl's action

The substantia nigra takes its name, which means "dark substance," from coloration caused by deposits of a pigment called neuromelanin. This compound, related to the skin pigment known as melanin, is thought to be the product of free radical activity and the substantia nigra's efforts to fight it.

Changes that occur over time in the neuromelanin deposits of the substantia nigra are sometimes considered to be a marker of physiological aging. Deprenyl has been shown to prevent these age-related changes. This effect could be taken as a further indication that deprenyl reduces both free radical activity and the rate of aging in this area of the brain [Knoll, 1986].

Unlike PEA and many of its close chemical relatives (including tyramine, amphetamine, and methamphetamine), deprenyl does not

"Increased concentration, energy and stamina, as a result an ability to cope with what would usually be difficult situations. Enhanced confidence as a result."
—One man describing his response to deprenyl
in *Smart Drugs II: The Next Generation*

displace catecholamines from their storage sites. Therefore it does not directly trigger catecholamine release and does not instigate an immediate increase in dopamine (or norepinephrine) activity. Rather, catecholamine activity builds up in response to deprenyl (over a nonetheless rather short time) through MAO B inhibition and uptake-blocking activity, as well as through other mechanisms not yet understood.

If deprenyl *did* trigger catecholamine release like other members of its chemical family, the benefits of its tyramine-uptake-blocking property (crucial to protection from the cheese effect) might be cancelled out to some degree. The conspicuous *absence* of catecholamine release effect may therefore constitute a third factor (along with selective MAO B inhibition and tyramine uptake blocking) contributing to deprenyl's unique safety [Knoll, 1992]. In sum, it seems that *three distinct properties* may be required to fully safeguard deprenyl from the possibility of hypertensive crisis—underscoring again the remarkable synergy of this compound's seemingly disparate effects.

## Deprenyl's Subjective Effects

Many people find that even a relatively small, single dose of deprenyl (five milligrams or less) can effect a subtle but distinct—and quite pleasant—change in their overall state of being. This has been described as "a mild-to moderate anti-depressant effect, increased energy, improved feelings of well-being, substantially increased sex drive, and more assertiveness" that "can last for several days" [Dean, 1993].

While the alteration of consciousness produced by commonly-used doses of deprenyl is probably not intense enough to be called a "high," some of those familiar with amphetamines have said that deprenyl's effects are similar (although lacking in the "edge" or tension often associated with these powerful stimulants).

Very high doses of deprenyl *have* produced unpleasant, amphetamine-like effects in some people. For further information, see the section on "Safety Issues."

## Deprenyl and Parkinson's

Deprenyl has been such a boon to the treatment of Parkinson's that it has been called "a miracle for many patients" [Fowkes, 1993]. While deprenyl is usually used in conjunction with L-dopa, some believe deprenyl may be on its way to replacing L-dopa as the treatment of choice for this condition [Dean, 1993].

Deprenyl's benefits in this arena are manifold. Foremost among them is the fact that deprenyl slows the progression of Parkinson's disease by forty to eighty-three per cent. As a result, Parkinson's patients using deprenyl in addition to standard therapy can expect to live about *two years longer* than those receiving standard treatment alone. Even *advanced* Parkinson's patients to whose regimen deprenyl is added, live significantly longer.

As explained in the chapter on L-dopa, standard therapy for Parkinson's consists of L-dopa, often with an additional compound for helping the body make more efficient use of this amino acid. While L-dopa does ameliorate Parkinsonian symptoms, it has, unlike deprenyl, no effect on the overall progression of the disease and does not extend the lives of Parkinson's patients [Knoll, 1983A].

When Parkinson's therapy begins with deprenyl instead of L-dopa, the need for L-dopa is significantly delayed. Furthermore, the concomitant use of deprenyl with L-dopa decreases the amount of L-dopa that is required by about twenty percent, thereby affording a reduction of L-dopa-related adverse effects. And some Parkinson's patients who start their therapy with deprenyl alone apparently *never* require L-dopa [Dilman, 1992; Fowkes, 1994; Dean, 1993].

Deprenyl not only *extends* life for Parkinson's patients, but enhances *quality* of life as well. Deprenyl treatment is associated with improved "alertness, drive, and motivation" in those suffering

"Deprenyl can often spectacularly improve the quality of the Parkinson's patient's life... An elderly man was so paralyzed by Parkinsonism that he was confined to his hospital bed, and his physician estimated that he had less than six months to live. His son got him into a wheel chair, and took him to a clinic in Switzerland. After a few weeks on deprenyl, the elderly gentleman had regained his faculties to a remarkable extent. He flew home with a five year supply. He soon resumed driving his own car and living alone in his own home. Within a few months he had three regular girlfriends! Before he ran out, he returned to Switzerland for another five year supply. He continued to be the neighborhood stallion for another four or five years, after which he no longer had the funds to fly back to Switzerland for a new supply. Within one week after running out, he was in the hospital. He died five weeks later."
— Durk Pearson and Sandy Shaw [1988]

(Note: Pearson and Shaw emphasize that this case is "not necessarily typical." Furthermore, it should be understood that the extraordinary effort required for this man to obtain deprenyl was caused by the absence of government approval for this medicine in the United States. Fortunately, the FDA has since approved deprenyl for the treatment of Parkinson's disease.)

from Parkinson's as well as "subjective feelings of increased vitality, euphoria, and increased energy" (effects typical of dopamine stimulation) [Dilman, 1992; Dean, 1993]. And, as detailed below in the section on "Deprenyl and Cognition," this drug has been demonstrated to improve several parameters of mental acuity in Parkinson's patients.

### Parkinson's, motor control, and deprenyl

Parkinson's disease was once known as "the shaking palsy." This phrase refers to the high-speed body tremors that are the most visible and obvious sign of Parkinson's. This shaking is part of the overall loss of motor control that characterizes Parkinson's.

As mentioned elsewhere in this book, dopamine plays an important role in motor function. This is especially true of dopamine in the striatum, an area of the brain discussed earlier in this chapter as a prime beneficiary of deprenyl's various effects. Striatal dopamine holds in check the amount of the neurotransmitter acetylcholine released by the caudate nucleus (a part of the striatum). Excessive levels of acetylcholine, a stimulant of motor activity, have been linked with Parkinson's symptoms. As dopamine levels in the caudate nucleus go down—as in aging and Parkinson's—acetylcholine levels tend to rise.

One way that deprenyl decreases Parkinson's symptoms is by boosting dopamine levels in the caudate nucleus, thereby limiting acetylcholine release. Another relevant mode of action may be the blocking of 6-OHDA uptake into dopamine neurons. (6-OHDA was discussed earlier as a naturally-occurring, toxic metabolite of dopamine that probably contributes to the development of Parkinson's.) Acetylcholine release approximately doubles in rats treated with 6-OHDA. However, levels of this neurotransmitter remain stable if the rats are given deprenyl one half-hour before 6-OHDA is administered [Knoll, 1986].

### Parkinson's, aging, and deprenyl

The loss of dopamine in the caudate nucleus has been correlated with both normal aging and the progression of Parkinson's disease. Dopamine content in this area of the brain tends to decrease by about thirteen percent per decade starting around the age of forty-five. When the dopamine content of the caudate nucleus falls below thirty percent of youthful levels, Parkinson's symptoms occur. A person in whom the dopamine level of this brain region has slipped below ten percent is considered "pre-morbid"—that is, near death [Knoll, 1992].

Taken together, these figures suggest that most people would begin to develop Parkinsonism around the age of ninety-five—if they lived that long. Joseph Knoll uses this kind of projection to argue that Parkinson's disease has no cause other than the aging of the striatal dopamine system. (In other words, it is not caused by a specific factor such as exposure to an MPTP-like toxin). Rather, he asserts, Parkinson's disease simply occurs in that segment of the population in whom this brain network happens to age the most rapidly [Knoll, 1992].

Life expectancy in our society has been steadily increasing for decades. It is likely that this trend will continue. If so, and if most people really would develop Parkinson's if they lived long enough, it follows that Parkinson's disease (which presently occurs in only one tenth of a percent of the population) will afflict growing numbers of people as time passes.

Not only is deprenyl of great benefit to those who already have Parkinson's disease; there is a strong probability that this compound will prove effective in *preventing* this condition. Given these attributes of deprenyl and the predictions about Parkinsonism and lifespan outlined above, it appears that deprenyl will very likely become an increasingly widely-used and vitally important medication in the future.

In fact, Knoll argues convincingly that virtually *everyone* should take deprenyl starting from the age of forty-five, not only for general life extension purposes but for the specific prevention of age-related neurological conditions such as Parkinson's and Alzheimer's.

## Deprenyl and Alzheimer's

Deprenyl has been called "a powerful new weapon against Alzheimer's disease" [Dean, 1993]. In numerous studies, deprenyl has significantly improved the performance of Alzheimer's patients. Furthermore, it has generally proven superior when tested against other drugs used for this condition [Dean, 1993; Knoll, 1992].

Deprenyl benefits Alzheimer's patients by heightening cognitive and verbal capacities, the early and rapid deterioration of which characterizes this disease. In one study, patients given only five milligrams of deprenyl per day for two months showed progress in verbal ability, attention, and memory, while those treated with placebo actually *lost* ground in these departments over the same time period.

A controlled study of verbal memory demonstrated significant improvement among Alzheimer's patients administered deprenyl for six months, as well as increased ability to use and apply new information the moment it is acquired. In other studies with Alzheimer's patients, deprenyl has benefitted short- and long-term memory, visuospatial ability, and prolonged concentration [Dean, 1993].

Joseph Knoll strongly recommends that deprenyl therapy be started immediately at the first indication that Alzheimer's disease is developing. Cutting-edge research is currently underway to further explore the application of deprenyl in the treatment of this condition [Fowkes, 1993].

## Deprenyl and Depression

MAO inhibitors have traditionally been considered of special value in treating certain kinds of atypical and suicidal depression that do not respond well to other forms of medication. The *Manual of Clinical Psychopharmacology* reports that deprenyl has demonstrated "a clear therapeutic effect in both atypical and endogenously [biochemically] depressed patients," and predicts that it "may turn out to be the best of the MAOIs—with fewer side effects and less risk of hypertensive crisis" than the older MAO inhibitors

[Schatzberg, 1990].

Not surprisingly, the manual notes that deprenyl also differs from other clinically-used MAOIs in that it "does not appear to cause...sexual dysfunction." Deprenyl may well, in fact, find a special niche as a prosexual alternative for people who have become frustrated by the negative sexual side effects of many commonly used antidepressants. Prozac, for example, while presently enjoying unprecedented popularity, is becoming well-known for markedly diminishing libido in both sexes. A man in his early forties interviewed for this book testifies that Prozac has been enormously helpful for relieving his depression; he complains, however, that "it has just about completely wiped out my sex drive." For this reason alone—and despite the tremendous benefits he has experienced—he plans to give up Prozac and seek an alternative.

> "I feel like I must have had a deprenyl deficiency all my life. Now I have energy and ambition. I feel like I've always thought other people must feel."
> —Thirty-four year-old woman

When used by itself in doses of fifteen to sixty milligrams a day, deprenyl is effective in relieving depression for about fifty percent of those treated [Schatzberg, 1990]. (This is a fairly typical response rate for an antidepressant). Unfortunately, this dosage range probably entails a risk of hypertensive crisis.

Fortunately, there is impressive evidence that the dosages of deprenyl required to treat depression can be substantially reduced by the addition of phenylalanine. Available as an over-the-counter supplement in health-food stores, phenylalanine is an amino acid used by the body to manufacture dopamine and norepinephrine, the same brain chemicals whose active levels are increased by deprenyl.

A European study of 155 depressed patients produced outstanding results through the daily administration of 250 milligrams of phenylalanine in conjunction with only five to ten milligrams of deprenyl [Dean, 1993]. Nearly seventy percent of the patients achieved total alleviation of depression, while more than twenty percent of the remaining patients exhibited "moderate improvement."

The treatment was well-tolerated by ninety percent of the subjects.

Comparable results were obtained in a much smaller study conducted in Chicago [Dean, 1993]. Only five milligrams of deprenyl, 100 milligrams of vitamin B-6, and one to six grams of phenylalanine were given every day to ten patients suffering from various types of major depression that had proved resistant to other drug therapies. Sixty percent of these patients reported *complete relief from depression* in only *two to three days*, whereas most antidepressants require *four to six weeks* for full effect.

The level of success achieved in these early studies represents a quantum leap in drug therapy for depression. Further results of this kind would firmly establish the deprenyl-plus-phenylalanine approach in a class by itself. (Furthermore, the doses of deprenyl allowed by this combination are far below levels at which the cheese effect becomes an issue.) Only electroshock therapy—a rather uninviting option for most—has demonstrated equal efficacy [Dean, 1993].

The people used in studies testing deprenyl's potency as an antidepressant had been diagnosed as "clinically," or severely, depressed. People who are only mildly or occasionally depressed, on the other hand, may find the smaller doses of deprenyl used for life-extension and prosexual purposes more than adequate for improving mood and providing extra "get-up-and-go." (See the "Dosages" section for further information.)

## Deprenyl and Cognition

As mentioned earlier, deprenyl improves various aspects of cognition in cases of Parkinsonism. In several studies conducted with Parkinson's patients, deprenyl has been shown to benefit memory, attention, and reaction times [Dilman, 1992; Dean, 1993]. And deprenyl's many boons to the mental function of those with Alzheimer's disease have just been discussed.

Deprenyl has been shown to affect positively the cognitive performance of normal, healthy animals [Dean, 1993]. In an eighteen-month study of rats identified as poor learners, animals maintained on deprenyl came to demonstrate much greater learning abilities than those treated with placebo [Knoll, 1992]. Maintenance on deprenyl also slows the normal, age-related loss of memory and learning ability in rats [Knoll, 1992].

Joseph Knoll has called deprenyl an "acute psychostimulant," indicating that a single dose of deprenyl can result in short-term stimulation of mental activity. As with the generalized mood elevation described earlier under "Deprenyl's Subjective Effects," many who have used deprenyl find that one dose of five milligrams,

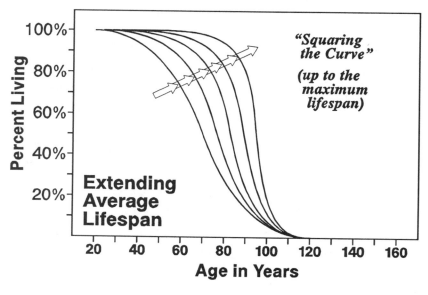

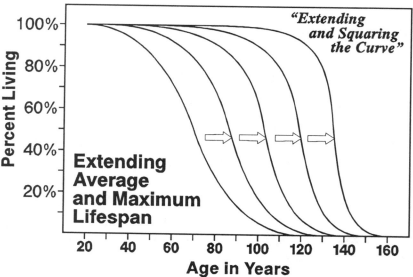

or even less, is sufficient to provide several hours of increased concentration, alertness, and mental stamina.

## Deprenyl and Life Extension

In the late 'eighties, Knoll and his colleagues published the results of a major study of deprenyl's life-extending effects in animals. This brilliantly constructed and carefully controlled series of experiments yield historical breakthroughs in two major areas of human and scientific endeavor: pharmacology and life extension.

The breakthrough nature of deprenyl's life extending effects hinges on the contrast between "maximum lifespan" and "average lifespan." The phrase "average lifespan" has the same meaning as the commonly-used phrase "normal life expectancy." In human beings, average lifespan is in the range of seventy to eighty years.

*Maximum* lifespan, on the other hand, is based on the idea of a built-in biological limit to potential lifespan. For human beings, maximum lifespan is thought to fall in the range of 115 to 120 years.

A number of substances—for instance, vitamin E and L-dopa—have been shown to increase the average lifespan of experimental animals. A technique that increases average lifespan allows greater numbers of a species to approach their maximum lifespan.

In a much celebrated experiment, Knoll and his colleagues tracked the longevity of one hundred thirty-two male rats. When the study started, these animals were two years old—the equivalent of early middle age for a human male. A control group consisting of half of these rats were administered placebo. The other half were placed on a program of continuous, low-dose administration of deprenyl (the same regimen found to maximize the facilitation of male rat sexual activity, as explained in the section "Deprenyl and Sex" below).

The average lifespan of the placebo-treated rats in this experiment turned out to be about one-hundred forty-seven weeks. The average lifespan of the deprenyl-treated group was about one-hundred ninety-one weeks. This result represents a *thirty percent increase in the average lifespan* for this group. An equivalent effect among humans would increase average lifespan to *just under one hundred years*.

This experimental demonstration of deprenyl's unrivaled efficacy in extending average lifespan, however, was accompanied by an even more impressive—and utterly unexpected—result.

All members of the placebo group were dead several weeks before the very first deprenyl-treated rat expired. In fact, the vast majority of those rats treated with deprenyl exceeded maximum lifespan for their species—in other words, they *lived longer than rats are supposed to be able to live*.

In an interview in *Mondo 2000* magazine, gerontologist Ward Dean M.D. encapsulated the historical significance of this result: "This is the first time that the maximum lifespan of any species has been extended through pharmacologic means."

The longest-lived animal in the control group reached one-hundred sixty-four weeks of age. The longest-lived rat in the deprenyl-treated group, however, reached nearly *two-hundred twenty six weeks*. Since the maximum lifespan of the rodent species used in these tests had previously been set at *only one hundred eighty-two weeks*, this result represents a *forty percent increase in maximum lifespan*. An equivalent effect in human beings would result in a maximum lifespan of approximately *one hundred seventy years* [Knoll, 1989; Dean, 1993].

An independent research group has verified the results of Knoll's experiment, producing similar effects in aging males of another rat species [Knoll, 1992].

In Knoll's longevity study, all animals were rated according to their level of sexual activity as displayed at the outset of the experiment. There was a clear correlation between sexual activity and lifespan among both the placebo group and the deprenyl group: the more sexually active the rats were, they longer they tended to live. This observation underscores a major theme of this book—the close relationship between longevity and sexual health.

### But what about humans?

Does deprenyl's miraculous life extending property—measured so far only in animals—extend to human beings as well?

A definitive answer to this question would require a marathon controlled study spanning several decades. However, the arguments favoring a similar effect among human beings—in the absence of credible cases to the contrary—have inspired a general consensus of confidence on the subject within the usually conservative pharmacological research community.

A persuasive case that deprenyl has a life-extending property in healthy human beings is offered by Joseph Knoll. He holds that studies of deprenyl's benefits for Parkinson's patients provide "convincing proof that the effects of [deprenyl] in humans are essentially similar to the ones found in our rat experiments" [Knoll, 1992].

The logic supporting this statement breaks down into five basic steps. Knoll begins with: 1) the rate at which deprenyl delays the need for L-dopa in Parkinson's therapy, and 2) the degree to which it extends the lives of Parkinson's patients. He combines this information with: 3) results from animal studies. He uses these statistics to calculate: 4) the rate at which

> "...progress may well include...drugs that change things we thought were irreversible."
> —Peter Kramer, M.D.
> author of *Listening to Prozac*

deprenyl slows the aging of the striatal dopamine system. Intentionally *undervaluing* the protective effect of deprenyl when projecting the resultant data to healthy people, Knoll uses this last figure to predict: 5) the numbers of years by which deprenyl is likely to extend both average and maximum lifespan in humans.

The conservative estimate produced by this method presumes that deprenyl will create only a small change in the rate of striatal dopamine loss—from thirteen percent to ten percent per decade—after the age of forty-five. Nonetheless, the final result is still at least a *fifteen-year extension of average lifespan* and a *thirty year extension of maximum lifespan* [Knoll, 1992].

### *More good news for human life-extenders*

*The Neuroendocrine Theory of Aging and Degenerative Disease*—a definitive, cutting-edge text on the process of aging—offers further encouragement for those pursuing life extension. Authors Dilman and Dean offer further support for the expectation that deprenyl will prove to slow aging in human beings.

Dilman and Dean report that deprenyl has been demonstrated to restore the sensitivity of a brain region called the hypothalamus to important biochemical signals from the rest of the body. The hypothalamus is widely regarded as the brain's chief center of management for the body's immune and endocrine functions. This organ is charged with maintaining the overall hormonal and chemical equilibrium that is technically known as "homeostasis." (For more detail, refer to the section of this book entitled "Some Basic Physiology.")

With aging, however, the dopamine-fuelled hypothalamus becomes less responsive to the biochemical fluctuations that it regulates. In Dilman and Dean's theory, the age-related loss of hypothalamic sensitivity plays a central, causal role in many of the processes that constitute normal aging.

"... our own personal experience with...deprenyl confirms that it is an aphrodisiac"—
Pearson & Shaw [1988]

Compounds such as L-dopa and deprenyl are key to Dilman and Dean's life extension strategy because they allow the hypothalamus to tune back in to the biochemical fluctuations that stimulate its proper functioning. Dilman and Dean also suggest that deprenyl may help to reverse age-related loss of immune function.

## Deprenyl and Sex

As mentioned in the chapter on L-dopa, Ward Dean MD, a pioneering physician in the area of life extension, has remarked that deprenyl is one of the compounds used regularly in his practice that patients most frequently comment upon in regard to strong prosexual qualities. Although prosexual results from deprenyl are probably most dramatic in men over 50 years old [Dean, 1993], this chemical is nonetheless developing a reputation for consistently enhancing sex and libido among both men and women of a broad age range— including those who consider themselves sexually vigorous and healthy to begin with.

Known primarily for increasing libido, the range of prosexual effects attributed to deprenyl seems to become broader as anecdotal evidence accumulates. For instance, a very sexually active 40-year-old single mother is convinced that deprenyl makes her "more lubricous" (meaning that her vagina becomes wetter)—an effect that, as far as we know, has not previously been documented.

In the following testimonial from a twenty-eight year-old male, deprenyl seems to exert a libidogenic power approaching that of the mythic "love potion." Here, if deprenyl did not in fact engender desire where *none* had previously existed—as the love potions of yore were believed to do—then at least this compound appears to have pushed it across a critical threshold:

> *"I remember taking deprenyl with a friend that I'd known for at least a year. Nothing sexual had ever happened between us. After a couple of hours of intense, intimate, and fun conversation we ended up taking off some of our clothes and 'making out' and cuddling. Nothing 'heavy,' mind you, but very pleasurable. I still hang out with her, and it's interesting to me that nothing like this ever happened between us before and hasn't since. In other words, the only time we ever got even slightly physical was also the only time we ever took deprenyl together."*

One forty-year-old male software entrepreneur even found deprenyl's effect on his libido "almost too hot to handle." He started to experiment with ten milligrams of deprenyl per day, primarily for relief of depression. "Deprenyl infused my sexuality with an aggressive quality," he says. "In fact, it was *too aggressive* for my taste." Although this effect dissipated to some degree over the period of usage, he ultimately abandoned deprenyl in favor of Prozac for treating depression.

This man's decision to switch illustrates the important role played by individual values and circumstances in determining whether a given pharmacological effect is positive or negative—especially when it comes to sexuality. When interviewed regarding the qualities that compose his personal definition of "better sex," this man emphasized intimacy, heart-connection, and emotional sensitivity.

"I already have a high 'baseline' sex drive," he explains, "which sometimes interferes with keeping my attention as focussed as it needs to be on the demands of my growing business. Partly due to this business aspect of my current life situation, there's not that much presently available to me in terms of sexual outlets anyway. And when I *do* have sex, I generally like it to be tender and gentle. Because of all these factors, I actually find Prozac's libido-dampening quality *desirable* in comparison to being aggressively horny from deprenyl."

The journal *Medical Aspects of Human Sexuality* has reported that "there are several ongoing studies examining the effects of deprenyl on sexual function." The anecdotal evidence sampled here predicts that this research will find deprenyl's prosexual effect among human beings comparable to that already demonstrated among animals. And, as the following section shows, deprenyl's enhancement of animal libido is quite impressive.

### Rat races

Between 1981 and 1992, Joseph Knoll and a small group of colleagues published at least eight scientific papers devoted to deprenyl's aphrodisiac properties in rats, often comparing it to other substances (among them apomorphine, bromocriptine, amphetamine, pargyline, and clorgyline). The results they have reported can be described as truly spectacular [Dallo, 1990; Yen, 1982; Knoll, 1983B; Dallo, 1992; Knoll, 1989; Dallo, 1986].

One of their articles is entitled "The Long Lasting, True Aphrodisiac Effect of Deprenyl in Sexually Sluggish Old Male Rats." As discussed elsewhere in this book, the scientific community has been reluctant to attribute *any* substances with "aphrodisiac" effects, and has, even in the last few decades, usually clung to the proposition that true aphrodisiacs have yet to be discovered. It is therefore significant in itself that Knoll and colleagues were confident enough in their results to risk using the words "long lasting, true aphrodisiac effect" not only in the *text* but in the actual *title* of the paper.

The methodology for determining the potency of aphrodisiac effects involved dividing the sexual behavior of male rats into three

Scientific research into sexuality isn't always a very sexy proposition. It's hard to imagine a less erotic scenario than a bunch of guys standing around in lab coats with clipboards observing "sexually sluggish old male rats" as they "mount, intromit, and ejaculate" in response to "receptive females" used as "stimulus objects."

Here's some more "hot 'n' heavy" research lingo used by Knoll and colleagues for describing the way they determined and quantified deprenyl's "aphrodisiac effects" in the report summarized in this chapter:

> indicator male
> non-copulators
> mount latency
> intromission latency
> ejaculation latency
> post-ejaculation interval
> mount frequency
> intromission frequency
> mean intromission interval
> ejaculation frequency
> mean ejaculation interval [Knoll, 1983B]

If you're still "in the mood" after reading *that* list, please notify the authors of this book. We suspect you've taken a *very* potent prosexual drug, and we want to hear about it.

stages: mounting, intromission (achievement of intercourse), and ejaculation. According to these standards of measurement, peak sexual vigor was represented by completion of this cycle with maximum frequency. Rats were divided into various experimental groups according to their level of sexual vigor prior to drug administration, which was also measured according to this continuum. (For example, some rats displayed no sexual behavior at all, others mounted with varying frequency but failed to achieve "intromission," and yet others achieved intromission but not ejaculation, etc.)

"Unfortunately, the bulk of existing literature is based upon studies of sexual behavior in rodents, the relevance of which to human sexuality is presently uncertain..."
—Rosen and Ashton [1993]

A dramatic and rather long-lasting effect was observed in response to a *single, low dose* of deprenyl injected underneath the skin of male rats considered "sexually sluggish" according to the standards described above. *Every single one* of a group of rats who had achieved *no ejaculations* in weekly "mating tests" for four consecutive weeks before receiving deprenyl achieved ejaculation in the test given one week after deprenyl was administered. In fact, all but two of the rats had *multiple ejaculations* in this test. Furthermore, *most of these rats continued to achieve ejaculation for the next three weeks*, and one managed to complete the mating act in this manner *five weeks after the low dose of deprenyl was administered*. (It is interesting to note that deprenyl's aphrodisiac effects in this experiment were somewhat delayed: none of the nine rats ejaculated in the mating test performed just twenty-four hours after the administration of deprenyl.)

Deprenyl was also effective in quickening the return to sexual activity of rats who had been "sexually exhausted," and in every type of test far surpassed the other compounds used for comparison (for instance, clorgyline and amphetamine).

A program of low doses of deprenyl—one quarter of a milligram per kilogram of body weight—administered three times a week on a long-term basis was found to produce the most potent prosexual effects. On this regimen, rats who had formerly been "sexually sluggish" maintained "full-scale sexual activity...in the long run." This program also stimulated at least some sexual activity for a period of several weeks in about half of the "non-copulators"— rats who had previously shown *no sexual behavior at all* (not even mounting).

Perhaps the most remarkable result of the entire series of experiments occurred when a group of "sexually sluggish, old male rats" (let's call them "geezers") on this program were compared with a group of sexually active younger males (let's call these rats "whippersnappers"). In this test, sexual activity was rated according to the percentage of rats in each group who achieved ejaculation in the weekly mating tests. In four weeks, the sexual activity of the geezers not only *caught up with* but *outstripped* that of the whippersnappers. In fact, the geezers roughly *doubled* the ejaculation percentages of the whippersnappers for the final four weeks of the test.

Knoll and colleagues concluded that their study had demonstrated the "remarkable efficacy" of deprenyl for "restoring and maintaining full-scale sexual activity" in geezer rats, who "maintained durably a level of sexual activity the height of which was comparable to the top performance of the [whippersnappers]." These results were apparently impressive enough to convince *even medical research scientists* that deprenyl exerted a "long lasting, true aphrodisiac effect" among the rats in question [Knoll, 1983B].

## Safety Issues

Deprenyl has maintained a good track record for safety in Europe for well over twenty years [Pearson, 1988]. The dosage required to inhibit MAO B in animals is less than half of one percent of deprenyl's LD-50 (the dose that causes fatality in half of the animals who receive it). In terms of milligrams per kilogram of body weight, the dosage required to produce MAO B inhibition in human beings is only about a tenth of that required for animals [Knoll, 1983A; Dean, 1993]. This information suggests that the difference between effective and potentially harmful doses may be even greater for people than it is for animals. Taken together, these facts demonstrate a margin of safety for deprenyl that has been called "remarkable" [Knoll, 1983A].

### Avoiding the cheese effect

The dosage level at which deprenyl may begin to pose some threat of the cheese effect has not been precisely determined. Furthermore, it is possible that the critical threshold varies from person to person.

One scientific paper reports that "neither hypertensive reactions nor the need for any special dietary care were ever encountered during long term (2-8 years) daily administration" of deprenyl in doses ranging from five to twenty milligrams. One study found that even huge amounts of tyramine provoked no changes in the blood pressure of people on deprenyl. Another study found that up to two hundred milligrams of tyramine—a quantity unlikely to be encountered in dietary form—could be consumed before blood pressure would begin to rise. In yet another study, even higher doses of deprenyl "failed to increase sensitivity to intravenous tyramine, whereas moderate doses of standard [MAO] inhibitors increased it considerably" [Knoll, 1992].

According to one source, a mild hypertensive reaction has nonetheless been reported in a person taking only twenty milligrams of deprenyl per day [Schatzberg, 1990]. Another source claims that "this response is observed to some degree at the sixty milligram level" [Dean, 1993]. However, the *Physicians' Desk Reference*, which proposes that MAO A inhibition may begin in the range of thirty to forty milligrams per day, states flatly that "cheese reactions *have not been reported* in selegiline treated patients" (emphasis added) [PDR, 1994].

The very confusion surrounding this issue could be taken as a positive sign of deprenyl's relative safety from the cheese effect. However, with a potentially life-threatening phenomenon such as hypertensive crisis, a policy of "better safe than sorry" is definitely advisable.

One thing is certain: no cheese reactions have ever been reported in people taking ten milligrams of deprenyl or less on a daily basis. We recommend that you exceed this dosage level *only* under the close supervision of a physician experienced with administering MAO inhibitors and *only* if you follow the appropriate dietary guidelines (which can be found in the *Physicians' Desk Reference* at your local library). In the unlikely event that ten milligrams per day of deprenyl turns out to be insufficient for your purposes, we suggest that you try potentiating deprenyl's effects with phenylalanine (and, possibly, vitamin B-6 as well) before considering a larger dose.

Hypertensive crisis can be recognized by a sudden, intense headache that begins in the area at the back of the head where the base of the skull meets the top of the neck. The pain then gradually spreads up and over the top of the head into the forehead and perhaps even the eyes and sinuses. If you think you may be having a hypertensive crisis, report immediately to the nearest hospital emergency room.

### Side effects

Most of deprenyl's recorded side effects have occurred in studies of elderly people using this drug in conjunction with L-dopa for Parkinson's disease. Fairly small percentages of these individuals have sometimes reported effects such as (in order of frequency): nausea; dizziness, light headedness, and fainting; abdominal pain; confusion; hallucinations; dry mouth; vivid dreams; and headache. (A more extensive list can be found in the *Physicians' Desk Reference*.) Information from such studies is not necessarily of great relevance for relatively healthy people using smaller doses for life extension and sexual enhancement, among whom side effects from deprenyl are very rare.

The side effects most likely to be experienced with deprenyl are probably those which sometimes characterize dopamine stimulation: nausea, headache, dizziness, and possibly even vomiting. Such phenomena are usually transient, can usually be terminated by reducing dosage (sometimes only temporarily), and can generally be avoided by starting small and slowly increasing dosage over time (see the section on "Dosages.")

You will know that you have definitely been taking *too much* deprenyl if you start to experience side effects like those sometimes associated with amphetamines. These include: "...feeling over-amped, sexually overstimulated, nauseous, irritable, emotionally hypersensitive, and even 'detached' from [one's] surroundings... vivid dreams, nightmares, and insomnia" [Dean, 1993].

### Contraindications

Deprenyl should not be used with meperidine (commonly known as Demerol). This precaution may extend to other opiates and opiate-like drugs [PDR, 1994]. Deprenyl should not be used with milacemide, a cognition-enhancer that is metabolized by MAO B. Using deprenyl in conjunction with other MAO inhibitors may also present problems [Dean, 1993].

## Dosages

The dosage of deprenyl that is appropriate for you will depend on your age, your personal biochemistry, and the effects you desire to achieve. Deprenyl can be taken *very* safely in dosages up to ten milligrams a day [Knoll 1992; PDR, 1994]. The addition of phenylalanine with or without vitamin B-6 may drastically reduce the dosage required, at least for purposes of cognitive enhancement or combatting depression.

As with most dopaminergic drugs, it may be wise to begin with a conservative dose and work your way up over a period of days or weeks, backing down if signs of overstimulation occur. (The effects of excessive doses have been described in the "Safety Issues" section under "Side effects.")

Joseph Knoll recommends that healthy people use ten to fifteen milligrams of deprenyl per week beginning at the age of forty-five. The purpose of this regimen is to combat the loss of dopamine that comes with normal aging and to prevent age-related neurological diseases [Knoll, 1992]. In the form of two or three five milligram tablets per week, Knoll's program is widely followed by people of a broad age range who use deprenyl for life-extension and prosexual purposes.

Discovery Experimental manufactures a liquid solution of deprenyl that can be measured out with reasonable accuracy in doses as low as a single milligram. This company recommends fine-tuning the dosage of deprenyl in accordance with chronological age. This program is made more practical by the unusual form of Discovery Experimental's deprenyl product.

Remember that many people are able to achieve a short-term prosexual effect, as well as cognitive stimulation, with only a single dose of deprenyl in the range of five milligrams. A disciplined, continuous regimen, like those advocated by Knoll and Discovery Experimental, is not always necessary in order to enjoy at least some of deprenyl's benefits. Those in search of life extension and/or long-term sexual rejuvenation, of course, will need to pursue a regular program.

## Legality and Availability

Deprenyl is available by prescription in the United States under the trade name Eldepryl. (Other names for deprenyl include Jumex and Movergan.) While its only approved used in United States is the treatment of Parkinsonism, some physicians may be willing to prescribe it for other purposes, and there are no legal impediments to their doing so.

Deprenyl can also be obtained legally—without a prescription—from various overseas mail-order sources, as long as the quantity you order can reasonably be considered no more than a three-month personal supply. (Please note, however, that we still recommend that you work with your personal physician.)

## Physicians and Product Sources

Please note the tearout card at the front of this book where you will find instructions for getting our *Directory of Mail Order Pharmacies* and *Directory of Physicians*. These listings are updated monthly. (Please also read the 'Disclaimer' section at the front of this book.)

# Other Prosexual Substances

The small selection of drugs and nutrients covered so far encompasses only the tip of the prosexual iceberg. We have amassed more than enough research to fill second and third volumes of *Better Sex Through Chemistry*. This chapter briefly discusses a few of the prosexual drugs and nutrients that have not yet appeared in this book.

**Nitric oxide** (not to be confused with *nitrous oxide* or "laughing gas," the common dental anesthetic) was the first neurotransmitter known to exist in the body in the form of a gas. Recent research has attributed the action of nitric oxide with primary responsibility for the vasodilation and smooth muscle relaxation involved in male erection.

A compound that increases levels of nitric oxide in the body has been developed as a therapy for impotence. This substance is administered by way of skin patches that work according to the same principle as the nicotine patches used to help people give up cigarettes.

An injectable form of **human growth hormone** has been developed and is now available by prescription. (Its only approved use so far is the treatment of growth-hormone-deficient children.) In one widely publicized study, injections of growth hormone were given for six months to twelve men ranging from 61 to 81 years of age. In a report published by the prestigious *New England Journal of Medicine*, the researchers who conducted this experiment claimed that growth hormone treatment reduced the biological age of the subjects by ten to twenty years [Todd, 1993].

Lord Lee-Benner, M.D., a physician and researcher specializing in applications of human growth hormone, describes the prosexual effects of growth hormone treatment in aging men: "Over a period of time it increases sexual interest and potency, and definitely enhances sensuality. It restores the intensity of orgasm to more youthful levels. For older people it definitely makes a big difference—like night and day."

A fair amount of controversy surrounds the safety of growth hormone injections. Furthermore, the compound is at present too expensive for most people. (A year's worth of the treatment used in the study described above, for example, would cost around ten thousand dollars for one person). In the next decade or so, this situation may change considerably. Further research may better

"British neurologist Giles S. Brindley M.D., has always been considered something of an iconoclast, but few were prepared for his unorthodox demonstration at a 1983 convention of urologists.

"The venue was Las Vegas and the conference room was packed with urologists and researchers from around the world. While most of the presenters were dressed in formal attire, Dr. Brindley took the podium in a loose-fitting sweatsuit. He addressed his fellow scientists by presenting the preliminary results of an investigational drug that generated erections when injected into the penis. About 15 minutes into his presentation, Dr. Brindley commented that his penis was getting hard. Most of the audience snickered, brushing the comment off as an attention-getting tactic.

"Dr. Brindley called their bluff. Stepping from behind the podium, he lowered his sweatpants to display a massive, rock-hard erection produced by an injection of this new drug, papaverine. The doctor casually strolled among the first few rows, inviting the urologists to feel and examine the rigidity of his drug-induced erection."

—Gary M. Griffin
Aphrodisiacs for Men [1991]

establish the safety of growth hormone treatment; the cost for consumers may decrease considerably; and the compound may become available in an orally active form. Meanwhile, bromocriptine, L-dopa, GHB, arginine, and ornithine can be used by those interested in increasing their growth hormone levels.

Another hormone of interest is **vasopressin**, currently popular as a nasal spray used for short-term cognition enhancement. Anecdotal reports consistently claim that a few whiffs of vasopressin before sex can increase the intensity of orgasm. Vasopressin is a pituitary hormone that suppresses release of prolactin (also a pituitary hormone). The sex-negative properties of excessive prolactin levels have been discussed in the chapter on bromocriptine.

**Apomorphine,** a short-acting stimulant of the dopamine system, has demonstrated some efficacy in facilitating erection. At present, this compound has no approved clinical applications and is used only in scientific research [Rosen, 1993].

**Vasoactive intestinal peptide, prostaglandin E1** (both members of the body's natural chemical repertoire) and **papaverine** reliably produce erections in men. Unfortunately, in order to do so, they must first be *injected* directly into the penis. Long-term use can therefore result in the development of penile scar tissue [Griffin, 1991]. Furthermore, according to one scientific paper, "many patients experience the injection itself, and the resulting erection, as painful, frightening, or subjectively aversive" [Rosen, 1993]. More appealing means of administering these compounds may soon be available.

Certain psychiatric medications are presently being explored for prosexual effects. The May, 1994 issue of *Penthouse* reports the findings of a doctor who has been successfully using **Prozac** to treat premature ejaculation. The November, 1994 issue discusses current research on the use of **Zoloft** (a new antidepressant) and **Anafranil** (used to treat compulsive behavior) for the same purpose. All of these compounds stimulate the serotonin system. Increased serotonin activity tends to pacify the libido—an effect which may actually serve a prosexual function in men who climax more quickly than they would like.

Studies have been performed to investigate the libido-enhancing properties of an antidepressant called **Wellbutrin (buproprion).**

Wellbutrin is unusual among clinically-used antidepressants for the specificity with which it stimulates dopamine activity. In one study, Wellbutrin was found to increase "sexual desire and subjective ratings of sexual satisfaction in a heterogenous group of sexually dysfunctional patients" [Rosen, 1993].

Many women have reported increased sex drive from the use of **piracetam**. This popular smart drug, which helps the brain to make more efficient use of oxygen, is known for its remarkable lack of toxicity.

### Who nose what the future holds?

The prosexual drugs of the near future may well include synthetic human **pheromones**. When released by the bodies of animals, pheromones stimulate powerful sexual responses from other members of the same species. A male cat's incessant, desperate yowling, for instance, is triggered by pheromones exuding from the nearby body of a female cat in heat. In fact, these chemicals mediate almost *all* sexual and social interaction in many animal species: "In addition to their orchestration of sex, pheromones help animals identify relatives, mark territories, and communicate bad intentions" [Wright, 1994].

According to theory, animals don't actually *smell* or *taste* pheromones. Instead, pheromones are detected by a special sensory organ that is located within the olfactory apparatus but has its own separate nerve connections to the brain.

Until the last few years, scientific consensus has held that pheromonal exchange does not take place among human beings.

"I took two grams of piracetam and, after 30 minutes, I began to find my boyfriend much more sexually attractive...Since this experience I have taken piracetam every day for two months and every time, without fail, it has had the same effect. Piracetam has vastly improved my sex life."
— a testimonial from *Smart Drugs & Nutrients*

Recent breakthrough research, however, has provided strong evidence that a tiny organ positioned about three inches inside the human nose responds to pheromones released by other human beings.

The economic potential of this discovery has not escaped the attention of venture capitalists. A new pharmaceutical firm—devoted to developing air-soluble drugs that will take effect by means of this pheromone-detecting organ—has already been founded. And a perfume supposedly containing human pheromones is already on the market [Wright, 1994].

These developments may herald a future in which many prosexual drugs will not be consumed by people who want to enhance their own sex drive or sex function. Instead, they will be *worn* by people who want to stimulate the sexual appetites of *others*.

Will the flagging sex life of an aging couple be re-ignited when the woman dabs her wrist with a scentless perfume that replicates the pheromonal output of a young co-ed? Or when the graying man mists his chest with a concoction labelled "Pheromone of Tall, Dark, Youthful Stallion"? Will some people's desire for a variety of sexual partners find fulfillment within a monogamous relationship by means of a rotating schedule of pheromonal formulae?

The prospects are intriguing.

Whatever the future of prosexual drugs may hold, we hope that *your* future will be abundant with prosexual effects.

## Physicians and Product Sources

Please note the tearout card at the front of this book where you will find instructions for getting our *Directory of Mail Order Pharmacies* and *Directory of Physicians*. These listings are updated monthly. (Please also read the 'Disclaimer' section at the front of this book.)

# References

## Introduction

Gary P. What is love? *Time.* February 15th, 1993.

Rosen RC; Ashton AK. Prosexual drugs: Empirical status of the 'new aphrodisiacs.' *Archives of Sexual Behavior.* 22(6): p521-43, 1993.

## Some Basic Physiology

Buffum J. Pharmacosexology: The effects of drugs on sexual function, a review. *J of Psychoactive Drugs.* 14(1-2): p5-43, Jan-Jun, 1982.

Dilman V; Dean, W. *The Neuroendocrine Theory of Aging & Degenerative Disease.* Pensacola, FL: The Center for Bio-Gerontology, 1992.

Everitt, BJ; Fuxe K. Dopamine and sexual behavior in female rats. Effects of dopamine receptor agonists and sulpiride. *Neurosci Lett (Netherlands)* 4/3-4: p209-13, 1977.

Mellow-Whipkit L. Drugs for sex: Real aphrodisiacs. *Mondo 2000.* Spring, 1991.

Sodersten P; Hansen S; Eneroth P. Inhibition of sexual behavior in lactating rats. *J Endocrinol.* 99(2): p189-97, November 1983.

Weizman R; Weizman A; Levi J; Gura V; Zevin D; Maoz B; Wijsenbeek H; Ben David M. Sexual dysfunction associated with hyperprolactinemia in males and females undergoing hemodialysis. *Psychosom Med.* 45(3): p259-69, June 1983.

# Part I: Natural Substances

## Prosexual Nutrients

Alexander JW; Gottschlich MM. Nutritional immunomodulation in burn patients. *Crit Care Med.* 18(2 suppl): p149-53, 1990.

Anggard E. Nitric oxide: mediator, murderer, and medicine. *The Lancet.* 343: p1199-207, 1994.

Associated Press. Researchers find male sex trigger. San Jose *Mercury News.* 2F: July 17, 1992.

Burnett AL; Lowenstein CJ; Bredt DS; et al. Nitric oxide: a physiologic mediator of penile erection. *Science.* 257: p401-4, 1992.

Clemens LG; Dohanich GP; Witcher JA. Cholinergic influences on estrogen-dependent seual behavior in female rats. *J Comp Physiol Psychol.* 95: p763-70, 1981.

Clemens LG; Barr P; Dohanich GP. Cholinergic regulation of female sexual behavior in rats demonstrated by manipulation of endogenous acetylcholine. *Physiol Behav.* 45: p437-42, 1989.

Daley JM; Reynolds J; Thom A; et al. Immune and metabolic effects of arginine in the surgical patient. *Ann Surg.* 208: p512-23, 1988.

Drexler H; Zeiher AM; Meinzer K; Just H. Correction of endothelial dysfunction in coronary microcirculation of hypercholesterolaemic patients by L-arginine. *Lancet.* 338: p1546-50, 1991.

Freundlich N. Much ado about NO. *Harvard Health Letter.* 18: p6-8, 1993.

Graham S. *A Lecture to Young Men.* Providence, Rhode Island: Weeden and Cory, 1834.

Griffith RS; DeLong DC; Nelson JD. Relation of arginine-lysine antagonism to Herpes simplex growth in tissue. *Chemotherapy.* 27: p209-13, 1981.

Hellstrom WJ; Monga M; Wang R; et al. Penile erection in the primate: induction with nitric-oxide donors. *J Urol.* 151: p1723-7, 1994.

Hoffman M. A new role for gases: neurotransmission; the remarkable finding that nitric oxide carries nerve impulses initiates a novel concept of neurotransmission. *Science.* 252: p1788, 1991.

Howe JW. *Excessive Venery, Masturbation and Continence.* New York: EB Treat, 1887.

Keller DW; Polakoski KL. L-arginine stimulation of human sperm motility in vitro. *Biol Reprod.* 13: p154-7, 1975.

Kellogg JH. *Plain Facts for Old and Young: Embracing the Natural History and Hygiene of Organic Life.* Burlington, Iowa: IF Stegner & Co, 1888.

Knopf; Conn; Fajans; et al. Plasma growth hormone response to intravenous administration if amino acids. *J Clin Endocrinol.* 25: p1140-4, 1965.

Kolata G. Key signals of cells found to be common gas. *New York Times.* C1, 2 July 1991.

Mani SK; Allen JM; Rettori V; et al. Nitric oxide mediates sexual behavior in female rats. *Proc Natl Acad Sci.* 91: p6468-72, 1994.

Merimee et al. Arginine-initiated release of human growth hormone. *N Eng J Med* 280: p1434-8, 1969.

Palmer RMJ; Rees DD; Ashton DS; et al. L-arginine is the physiological precursor for the formation of nitric oxide in endothelium dependent relaxation. *Biochem Biophys Res Comm.* 153: p1251-6, 1988.

Papp G; Grof J; Molnar J; Jambor E. Die Rolle des Arginingehaltes und der Arginase-Aktivitat in der Fertilitat. *Andrologia.* 11: p37-41, 1979.

Pau MY; Milner JA. Dietary arginine and sexual maturation of the female rat. *J Nutr.* 112: p1834-42, 1982.

Pearson D; Shaw S. *The Life Extension Weight Loss Program.* New York: Doubleday & Co., 1986.

Pearson D; Shaw S. *The Life Extension Companion.* New York: Warner Books, 1984.

Pearson D; Shaw S. *Life Extension: A Practical Scientific Approach.* New York: Warner Books, 1982.

Pearson D; Shaw S. Sexual effects of nutrients: arginine and choline. *Lifenet News.* II: p6, 1991.

Ralli EP; Dunn SD. Relation of pantothenic acid to adrenal cortical function. *Vit Horm.* 11: p133-158, 1953.

Rudman D; Axel MD; Hoskote S; et al. Effects of human growth hormone in men over 60 years old. *N Engl J Med.* 323: p1-5, 1990.

Saito M; Broderick GA; Hypolite JA; Levin RM. Pharmacological effect of ethanol on the function of rabbit corporal cavernosal tissue. *Pharmacology.* 48: p335-40, 1994.

Salvadorini F.; Todeschini G.; Tognetti G.; Marescotti V. Effects of oral treatment with arginine in subjects affected by hypospermia. *Rass Int Clin Ter.* 54: p319-30, 1974.

Wang R; Domer FR; Sikka SC; et al. Nitric oxide mediates penile erection in cats. *J Urol.* 151: p234-7, 1994.

Wilson HR; Harms RH. Evaluation of nutrient specifications for broiler breeders. *Poult Sci.* 63: p1400-6, 1984.

Yallampalli C; Byam-Smith M; Nelson SO; Garfield RE. Steroid hormones modulate the production of nitric oxide and cGMP in the rat uterus. *Endocrinology.* 134: p1971-4, 1994.

## GHB (gamma-hydroxybutyrate)

Artru AA; Steen PA; Michenfelder JD. y-Hydroxybutyrate: Cerebral metabolic, vascular, and protective effects. *Journal of Neurochemistry.* 35(5): p1114-9, November 1980.

Cash, CD. Gammahydroxybutyrate: An overview of the pros and cons for it being a neurotransmitter and/or a useful therapeutic agent. *Neuroscience and Biobehavioral Reviews.* 18(2): p291-304, 1994.

Chin MY; Kreutzer RA; Dyer JE. Acute poisoning associated with gamma-hydroxybutyrate in California. *West J Med (UNITED STATES)*. 156(4): p380-4, Apr 1992. (California Department of Health Services, Environmental Epidemiology and Toxicology Branch, Emeryville 94608.)

Cooper, JR; Bloom, FE; Roth, RH. *The biochemical basis of neuropharmacology, 2nd edition*. New York, London, Toronto: Oxford University Press, 1974.

Dean W; Morgenthaler J; Fowkes S. *Smart Drugs II: The Next Generation*. Petaluma, California: Smart Publications, 1993.

Fadda F; Colombo G, Mosca E; Gessa GL. Suppression by gamma-hydroxybutyric acid of ethanol withdrawal syndrome in rats. *Alcohol & Alcoholism*. 24(5): p447-51, 1989. (Printed in Great Britain.)

Fowkes, S. Q&A. *Smart Drug News*. 2(2): March 1993. (CERI, POB 4029, Menlo Park, CA, 94026-4029, tel:415-321-2374, fax:415-323-3864)

Gallimberti L; Gentile N; Cibin M; Fadda F; Canton G; Ferri M; Ferrara SD; Gessa GL. Gamma-hydroxybutyric acid for treatment of alcohol withdrawal syndrome. *The Lancet*. p787-9, 30 September 1989.

Kleimenova NN; Ostrovskaya RU; Arefolov VA. Effect of sodium hydroxybutyrate on the ultrastructure of the cross-striated muscle tissue myocytes during physical exercise. *Byull Eksp Biol Med*. 88(9): p358-61, 1979. (Inst Pharmacol, Moscow USSR.)

Laborit H. Correlations between protein and serotonin synthesis during various activities of the central nervous system (slow and desynchronized sleep, learning and memory, sexual activity, morphine tolerance, aggressiveness, and pharmacological action of sodium gamma-hydroxybutyrate). *Research Communications in Chemical Pathology and Pharmacology*. 3(1): Jan 1972.

Laborit H. Sodium 4-hydroxybutyrate. *Int J Neuropharmacology*. 3: p433-52, 1964. (Pergamon Press. Printed in Great Britain.)

Ostrovskaya RU; Kleimenova NN; Kamisheva V; Molodavkin GM; Yavorskii AN; Boikko SS. Effect of sodium hydroxybutyrate on functional biochemical and morphological indexes of physical working ability. *Farmakol Regul Protsessov Utomleniya (Moscow USSR)*. 39(56): p112-17, 1982.

Pearson D; Shaw S. *Life Extension: A Practical Scientific Approach*. New York: Warner Books, 1982.

Pearson D; Shaw S. *Durk Pearson & Sandy Shaw's Life Extension Newsletter*. 2: October 1988.

Rogers P; Katel P. The new view from on high. *Newsweek*. 6 December 1993.

Takahara J; Yunoki S; Yakushiji W; Yamauchi J; Yamane J; Ofuji T. Stimulatory effects of gamma-hydroxybutyric acid on growth hormone and prolactin release in humans. *J Clin Endocrinal Metab*. 44: p1014, 1977.

Vickers MD. Gammahydroxybutyric acid. *Int Anaesthesia Clinic*. 7: p75-89, 1969.

Watson CM. *Love Potions: A Guide to Aphrodisiacs and Sexual Pleasures.* Tarcher/Perigee, 1993.


## L-Dopa

Angrist B; Gershon S. Clinical effects of amphetamine and L-dopa on sexuality and aggression. *Comprehenspsychiat (USA).* 17(6): p715-22, 1976.

Ballivet J; Marin A; Gisselmann A. [Aspects of the hypersexuality observed in the parkinsonian subject during treatment with levodopa.] Aspects de l'hypersexualite observee chez le parkinsonien lors du traitement par la L-dopa. *Annmed-Psychol (France).* 131(II/4): p515-22, 1973.

Barbeau A. Neurological and psychiatric side effects of L-dopa. *Pharmacol ther ser c (United Nations).* 1(3-4): p475-94, 1976.

Bianchine JR. Sexual function in Parkinson's disease. *Med Aspects Hum Sex (USA).* 13(4): p69-70, 1979.

Block, W. Affects of bromocriptine on the brain. *Life Extension Report.* 13(10): p75-8, October 1993.

Boyd et al. "Stimulation of human-growth-hormone secretion by L-dopa." *New Engl J Med.* 183(26): p1425-9, 1970.

Brown E; Brown GM; Kofman O; Quarrington B. Sexual function and affect in parkinsonian men treated with L-dopa. *Am J Psychiatry.* 135(12): p1552-5, Dec 1978.

Buffum J. Pharmacolsexology: The effects of drugs on sexual function, a review. *J of Psychoactive Drugs.* 14(1-2): p5-43, Jan-Jun, 1982.

Castaigne P. [Levodopa and mental disturbances.] L-dopa et troubles psychiques. *Int J Neurol (Montevideo) (Uruguay).* 10(1-4): p178-85, 1975.

Cotzias, GC; Miller, ST; Tang, LC; Papava siliou, PS; Wang, YY. "Levodopa, fertility and longevity." *Science.* 196: p549-551, 1977.

Dean W; Morgenthaler J; Fowkes S. *Smart Drugs II: The Next Generation.* Petaluma, California: Smart Publications, 1993.

Dilman V; Dean, W. *The Neuroendochrine Theory of Aging & Degenerative Disease.* Pensacola, FL: The Center for Bio-Gerontology, 1992.

Fowkes, S. Q&A. *Smart Drug News.* 2(10): Feb 1994. (CERI, POB 4029, Menlo Park, CA, 94026-4029, tel:415-321-2374, fax:415-323-3864)

Gawin FH. Drugs and eros: reflections on aphrodisiacs. *J Psychoative Drugs.* 10(3): p227-36, Jul-Sep 1979.

Girke W; Xenakis Ch. [Side effects of L-dopa treatment.] Nebenwirkungen der L-dopa therapie. *Dtsch Med Wschr (Germany, West).* 100(42): p2165-9, 1975.

Gray GD; Davis HN; Dewsbury DA. Effects of L-dopa on the heterosexual copulatory behavior of male rats. *Eur J Pharmacol (Amst) (Netherlands)*. 27(3): p367-70, 1974.

Keyes DM; Janzik HH; Mayer K; et al. L-dopa effects on sexual behaviour: an experimental study. *J Sex Res (USA)*. 12(2): p117-23, 1976.

Koller WC; Veter-Overfield B; Williamson A; Busenbark K; Nash J; Parrish D. Sexual dysfunction in Parkinson's disease. *Clin Neuropharmacol (USA)*. 13(5): p461-3, 1990.

Laborit H. Correlations between protein and serotonin synthesis during various activities of the central nervous system (slow and desynchronized sleep, learning and memory, sexual activity, morphine tolerance, aggressiveness, and pharmacological action of sodium gamma-hydroxybutyrate). *Research Communications in Chemical Pathology and Pharmacology*. 3(1): Jan 1972.

Malmnas CO. The significance of dopamine, versus other catecholamines, for L-dopa induced facilitation of sexual behavior in the castrated male rat. *Pharm Biochem Behav (USA)*. 4(5): p521-6, 1976.

Pearson D; Shaw S. *Life Extension: A Practical Scientific Approach* New York: Warner Books, 1982.

*Physicians' Desk Reference (PDR)*. Montvale, New Jersey: Medical Economics Data, a division of Medical Economics Company, Inc, 1994.

Quinn NP; Toone B; Lang AE; et al. Dopa dose-dependent sexual deviation. *Br J Psychiatry (England)*. 142(3): p296-8, 1983.

Ryan EL; Frankel AI. The effect of L-3,4-dihydroxyphenylalanine (L-dopa) on the prolactin response to sexual behavior in the male rat. *Neuroendocrinology (Switzerland)*. 28(5): p302-6, 1979.

Selby G. Laevodopa in Parkinson's disease: an Australian trial. *Neurology (Bombay) (India)*. 20(2 sup): p203-14, 1972.

Sietnieks A; Meyerson BJ. Enhancement by progesterone of 5-hydroxytryptophan inhibition of the copulatory response in the female rat. *Neuroendocrinology (Switzerland)*. 35(5): p321-6, 1982.

Singer C; Weiner WJ; Sanchez-Ramos JR. Autonomic dysfunction in men with Parkinson's disease. *Eur Neurol (Switzerland)*. 32(3): p134-40, 1992.

Tagliamonte A; Fratta W; Del Fiacco M; Gessa GL. Possible stimulatory role of brain dopamine in the copulatory behavior of male rats. *Pharm Biochem Behav (USA)*. 2(2): p257-60, 1974.

Uitti RJ; Tanner CM; Rajput AH; Goetz CG; Klawans HL; Thiessen B. Hypersexuality with antiparkinsonian therapy. *Clin Neuropharmacol*. 12(5): p375-83, Oct 1989.

Vogel HP; Schiffter R. Hypersexuality--a complication of dopaminergic therapy in Parkinson's disease. *Pharmacopsychiatria (Germany, West)*. 16(4): p107-10, Jul 1983.

## Yohimbe & Yohimbine

Adaikan PG; Ratnam SS. Pharmacology of penile erection in humans. *Cardiovasc Intervent Radiol.* 11(4): p191-4, 1988.

Bowes MP; Peters RH; Kernan WJ Jr; Hopper DL. Effects of yohimbine and idazoxan on motor behaviors in male rats. *Pharmacol Biochem Behav (USA),.* 41(4): p(707-13, 1992.

Buffum J. Pharmacosexology update) Yohimbine and sexual function. *J Psychoact Drugs (USA).* 17(2): p131-2, 1985.

Buffum J. Pharmacolsexology: The Effects of Drugs on Sexual Function, a Review. *J of Psychoactive Drugs.* 14(1-2): p5-43, Jan-Jun, 1982.

Clark JT. Suppression of copulatory behavior in male rats following central administration of clonidine. *Neuropharmacology (United Kingdom).* 30(4): p373-82, 1991.

Clark JT; Smith ER; Davidson JM. Testosterone is not required for the enhancement of sexual motivation by yohimbine. *Physiol Behav (USA).* 35(4): p517-21, 1985.

Clark JT; Smith ER; Davidson JM. Evidence for the modulation of sexual behavior by alpha-adrenoceptors in male rats. *Neuroendocrinology (Switzerland).* 41(1): p36-43, 1985.

Clark JT; Smith ER; Davidson JM. Enhancement of sexual motivation in male rats by yohimbine. *Science (United States).* 225(4664): p847-9, Aug 24 1984.

Costa R; Marino A. [On the eventual psychotropic, cardiovascular and aphrodisiac properties of yohimbine, an old drug with new indications.] Sulle eventuali proprieta psicotrope, cardioangioattive e afrodisiache della yoimbina, vecchio farmaco con nuove indicazioni. *Clin Ter (Italy).* 129(3): p159-68, May 15 1989.

Davis GA; Kohl R. The Influence of alpha receptors on lordosis in the female rat. *Pharm Biochem Behav (USA).* 6(1): p47-53 , 1977.

Deamer RL; Thompson JF. The role of medications in geriatric sexual function. *Clin Geriatr Med (USA).* 7(1): p95-111, 1991.

Dohler DD; Jarzab B; Sickmoller PM; Kokocinska D; Kaminski M; Gubala E; Achtelik W; Wagiel J. Influence of neurotransmitters on sexual differentiation of brain structure and function. *Exp Clin Endocrinol (Germany).* 98(2): p99-109, 1991.

Friesen K; Palatnik W; Tenenbein M. Benign course after massive ingestion of yohimbine. *J Emerg Med (United States).* 11(3): p287-8, May-Jun 1993.

Gawin FH. Drugs and eros: Reflections on aphrodisiacs. *J Psychoative Drugs.* 10(3): p227-36, Jul-Sep 1979.

Gottlieb A. *Sex Drugs and Aphrodisiacs.* 20th Century Alchemist, 1974.

Green J. *The Male Herbal: Health Care for Men and Boys.* Freedom, California: Crossing Press, 1991.

Griffin GM. *Aphrodisiacs For Men.* Added Dimensions Publishing, 1991.

Grossman E; Rosenthal T; Peleg E; Holmes C; Goldstein DS. Oral yohimbine increases blood pressure and sympathetic nervous outflow in hypertenseive patients. *Cardiovasc Pharmacol (United States).* 22(1): p22-6, Jul 1993.

Hollander E; McCarley A. Yohimbine treatment of sexual side effects induced by serotonin reuptake blockers. *J Clin Psychiatry (United States).* 53(6): p207-9, Jun 1992.

Jacobsen FM. Fluexotine-induced sexual dysfunction and an open trial of yohimbine. *J Clin Psychiatry (United States).* 53(4): p119-22, Apr 1992.

Laborit H. Correlations Between Protein and Serotonin Synthesis During Various Activities of the Central Nervous System (Slow and Desynchronized Sleep, Learning and Memory, Sexual Activity, Morphine Tolerance, Aggressiveness, and Pharmacological Action of Sodium Gamma-Hydroxybutyrate). *Research Communications in Chemical Pathology and Pharmacology.* 3(1): Jan 1972.

Lin SN; Yu PC; Yang MC; Chang LS; Chiang BN; Kuo JS. Local suppressive effect of clonidine on penile erection in the dog. *J Urol (United States).* 139(4): p849-52, Apr 1988.

Morales A; Condra M; Owen JA; Surridge DH; Fenemore J; Harris C. Is yohimbine effective in the treatment of organic impotence? Results of a controlled trial. *J Urol (United States).* 137(6): p1168-72, Jun 1987.

Morpurgo B; Rozenboim I; Robinzon B. Effect of yohimbine on the reproductive behavior of the male Nile crocodile Crocodylus nilicotus. *Pharmacol Biochem Behav (USA).* 43(2): p449-52, 1992.

Naumenko EV; Amstislavskaja TG; Osadchuk AV. The role of adrenoceptors in the activation of the hypothalamic-pituitary-testicular complex of mice induced by the presence of a female. *USSR Exp Clin Endocrinol (Germany).* 97(1): p1-11, 1991.

*Physicians' Desk Reference (PDR).* Montvale, New Jersey: Medical Economics Data, a division of Medical Economics Company, Inc., 1994.

Price J; Grunhaus LJ. Treatment of Clomipramine-induced anorgasmia with yohimbine: A case report. *J Clin Psychiatry (USA).* 51(1): p32-3, 1990.

Reid K; Surridge DH; Morales A; Condra M; Harris C; Owen J; Fenemore J. Double-blind trial of yohimbine in treatment of psychogenic impotence. *Lancet (England).* 2(8556): p241-3, 22 Aug 1987.

Richard Alan Miller. *The Magical and Ritual Use of Aphrodisiacs.* Destiny Books, 1985.

Rosen RC; Ashton AK. Prosexual Drugs: Empirical status of the 'new aphrodisiacs.' *Archives of Sexual Behavior.* 22(6): p521-43, 1993.

Sala M; Braida D; Leone MP; Calcaterra P; Monti S; Gori E. Central effect of yohimbine on sexual behavior in the rat. *Physiol Behav (USA).* 47(1): p165-73, 1990.

Smith ER; Davidson JM. Yohimbine attenuates aging-induced sexual deficiencies in male rats. *Physiol Behav (USA).* 47(4): p631-634, 1990.

Smith ER; Lee RL Schnur SL; Davidson JM. Alpha2-adrenoceptor antagonists and male sexual behavior: I Mating Behavior *Physiol Behav (USA)*. 41(1): p7-14, 1987A.

Smith ER; Lee RL Schnur SL; Davidson JM. Alpha2-adrenoceptor antagonists and male sexual behavior: II Erectile and ejaculatory reflexes. *Physiol Behav (USA)*. 41(1): p15-9, 1987B.

Sonda LP; Mazo R; Chancellor MB. The role of yohimbine in the treatment of erectile impotence. *J Sex Marital Ther (United States)*. 16(1): p15-21, Spring 1990.

Stafford, Peter. *Psychedelics Encyclopedia, 3rd Edition*. Ronin Press, 1993.

Susset JG; Tessier CD; Wincze J; Bansal S; Malhotra C; Schwacha MG. Effect of yohimbine hydrochloride on erectile impotence: a double-blind study. *J Urol (United States)*. 141(6): p1360-3, Jun 1989.

Watson CM. *Love Potions: A Guide to Aphrodisiacs and Sexual Pleasures*. Tarcher/Perigee, 1993.

Yates A; Wolman W. *Aphrodisiacs: Myth and Reality*. Medical Aspects of Human Sexuality. p58-61, December 1991.

Yonezawa A; Kawamura S; Ando R; Tadano T; Kisara K; Kimura Y. Chronic clonidine treatment and its termination: Effects on penile erection and ejaculation in the dog. *Life Sci. (USA)*. 51(25): p1999-2007, 1992.

# Part II: Synthetic Substances

## Bromocriptine

Andronova LM. [Possibilities for behavior correction in a learned ethanol preference in female and male white rats.] *Farmakol Toksikol*. 50(4): p55-60, Jul-Aug 1987.

Ayalon D; Eckstein N; Homonnai ZT; Paz GF; Eshel A; Reider. Effects of long-term treatment with bromocriptine on pituitary prolactinoma in a male. *I Int J Gynaecol Obstet*. 20(6): p481-5, Dec 1982.

Baas H.; Schneider E.; Fischer P.-A.; Japp G. Mesulergine and bromocriptine in long-term treatment of advanced parkinsonism. *West J Neural Transm. (Austria)*. 64(1): p45-54, 1985.

Bacz A.; Klimek R. Clinical evaluation of short-lasting administration of bromcriptine preparation in men. *Klin Endokrynol*. 50(10): p875-8, 1979.

Barnett PS; Palazidou E; Miell JP; Coskeran PB; Butler J; Dawson JM; Maccabe J; McGregor AM. Endocrine function, psychiatric and clinical consequences in patients with macro-prolactinomas after long-term treatment with the new non-ergot dopamine agonist CV205--502. *Q J Med* 81(295): p891-906, Nov 1991.

Bergh T.; Nillius J.; Wide L. Bromocriptine treatment of 42 hyperprolactinaemic women with secondary amenorrhoea. *Sweden Acta Endocrinol. (Copenhagen) (Denmark)*. 88(3): p435-51, 1978.

Besser GM; Wass JA; Thorner MO. Acromegaly--results of long term treatment with bromocriptine. *Acta Endocrinol Suppl (Copenh)*. 216: p187-98, 1978.

Blin O.; Schwertschlag U.S.; Serratrice G. Painful clitorial tumescence during bromocriptine therapy (25). *Lancet (United Kingdom)*. 337(8751): p1231-2, 1991.

Block, W. Affects of Bromocriptine on the Brain. *Life Extension Report*. 13(10): p75-8, October 1993.

Bommer, J; Ritz E; del Pozo E; Bommer G. Improved sexual function in male haemodialysis patients on bromocriptine. *Lancet*. 2(8141): p496-7, 8 Sep 1979.

Brown E; Brown GM; Kofman O; Quarrington B Am J. Sexual function and affect in parkinsonian men treated with L-dopa. *Psychiatry*. 135(12): p1552-5, Dec 1978.

Buffum J. Pharmacolsexology: The Effects of Drugs on Sexual Function, a Review. *J of Psychoactive Drugs*. 14(1-2): p5-43, Jan-Jun, 1982.

Buvat J; Lemaire A; Buvat-Herbaut M; Fourlinnie JC; Racadot A; Fossati P. Hyperprolactinemia and sexual function in men. *Horm Res*. 22(3): p196-203, 1985.

Ciccarelli E; Miola C; Grottoli S; Avataneo T; Lancranjan I; Camanni F. Long term therapy of patients with macroprolactinoma using repeatable injectable bromocriptine. *J Clin Endocrinol Metab (US)*. 76(2): p484-8, Feb 1993.

Cincotta AH; Meier AH. Reductions of body fat stores and total plasma cholesterol and triglyceride concentrations in several species by bromocriptine treatment. *Life Sciences* 45: p2247-54, 1989.

Clinical Research, Sandoz Limited, Basle Switzerland. The safety of bromocriptine in long-term use: A review of the literature. *Curr Med Res Opin. (UK)*. 10(1): p25-51, 1986.

Cocores JA; Dackis CA; Gold MS. Sexual dysfunction secondary to cocaine abuse in two patients. *J Clin Psychiatry*. 47(7): p384-5, Jul 1986.

Dallo J; Lekka N; Knoll J. The ejaculatory behavior of sexually sluggish male rats treated with (-)deprenyl, apomorphine, bromocriptine and amphetamine. *Pol J Pharmacol Pharm*. 38(3): p251-5, May-Jun 1986.

Deamer RL; Thompson JF. The role of medications in geriatric sexual function. University of California, Los Angeles School of Medicine. *Clin Geriatr Med*. 7(1): p95-111, Feb 1991.

Dean W; Morgenthaler J; Fowkes S. *Smart Drugs II: The Next Generation*. Petaluma, California: Smart Publications, 1993.

Dilman V; Dean, W. *The Neuroendochrine Theory of Aging & Degenerative Disease*. Pensacola, FL: The Center for Bio-Gerontology, 1992.

el-Beheiry A; Souka A; el-Kamshoushi A; Hussein S; el-Sabah K. Hyperprolactinemia and impotence. *Arch Androl*. 21(3): p211-4, 1988.

Ermolenko VM; Kukhtevich AV; Dedov II; Bunatian AF; Melnichenko GA; Gitel EP. Parlodel treatment of uremic hypogonadism in men. *Nephron*. 42(1): p19-22, 1986.

Everitt BJ. Monoamines and sexual behaviour in non-human primates. *Ciba Found Symp.* (62): p329-58, Mar 14-16 1978.

Eversmann T; Eichinger R; Fahlbusch R; Rjosk HK; von Werder K. [Hyperprolactinemia in the male: clinical aspects and therapy.] *Schweiz Med Wochenschr.* 111(47): p1782-9, 21 Nov 1981.

Foster R.S.; Mulcahy J.J.; Callaghan J.T.; Crabtree R.; Brashear D. Role of serum prolactin determination in evaluation of impotent patient. *Urology (USA).* 36(6): p499-501, 1990.

Grimes JD; Hassan MN. Bromocriptine in the long-term management of advanced Parkinson's disease. *Can J Neurol Sci (Canada).* 10(2): p86-90, 1983.

Huang et al, "Induction of estrous cycles in old non-cyclic rats by progesterone, ACTH, ether stree, or L-dopa." *Neuroendocrin.* 20: p21-34, 1976.

Julien, R. *A Primer of Drug Action*, 5th Edition. New York: W. H. Freeman and Company, 1988.

Kaliszuk S; Borzecki Z; Swies Z. The influence of bromocriptine on sexual activity in ethanol-exposed male rats. *Sklodowska [Med] (Poland).*44: p109-14, 1989.

Katzir D; Rosenberg T; Ramot Y; Gaver-Shavit A; Gilboa Y. [Treatment of prolactin-secreting pituitary tumors with bromocriptine.] *Harefuah.* 118(3): p141-5, Feb 1, 1990.

Kirby RW; Kotchen TA; Rees ED. Hyperprolactinemia--a review of recent clinical advances. *Arch Intern Med.* 139(12): p1415-9, Dec 1979.

Kocijancic A; Prezelj J; Vrhovec I; Lancranjan I. Parlodel LAR in the treatment of macroprolactinomas. *Acta Endocrinol (Copenh).* 122(2): p272-6, Feb 1990.

Koenig MP; Zuppinger K; Liechti B. Hyperprolactinemia as a cause of delayed puberty: successful treatment with bromocriptine. *J Clin Endocrinol Metab.* 45(4): p825-8, Oct 1977.

Konig MP; Kopp P. [Hyperprolactinemia.] *Schweiz Med Wochenschr.* 116(9): p265-70, Mar 1 1986.

Koppelman MC; Parry BL; Hamilton JA; Alagna SW; Loriaux DL. Effect of bromocriptine on affect and libido in hyperprolactinemia. *Am J Psychiatry.* 144(8): p1037-41, Aug 1987.

Lamberts SW; Quik RF. A comparison of the efficacy and safety of pergolide and bromocriptine in the treatment of hyperprolactinemia. *J Clin Endocrinol Metab.* 72(3): p635-41, Mar 1991.

Landolt AM; Froesch ER. [Prolactin producing hypophyseal adenoma: diagnosis and therapeutic possibilities.] *Schweiz Med Wochenschr.* 115(23): p803-9, 8 Jun 1985.

Martin-Du Pan R. [Neuroleptics and sexual dysfunction in man. Neuroendocrine aspects] *Schweiz Arch Neurol Neurochir Psychiatr.* 122(2): p285-313, 1978.

Mbanya J.-C.N.; Mendelow A.D.; Crawford P.J.; Hall K.; Dewar J.H.; Kendall-Taylor P. Rapid resolution of visual abnormalities with medical therapy alone in patients with large prolactinomas. *J Neurosurg. (United Kingdom).* 7(5:): p519-527, 1993.

Montini M; Pagani G; Gianola D; Pagani MD; Salmoiraghi M; Ferrari L; Lancranjan I. Long-lasting suppression of prolactin secretion and rapid shrinkage of prolactinomas after a long-acting, injectable form of bromocriptine. *J Clin Endocrinol Metab.* 63(1): p266-8, Jul 1986.

Moussa, 1985 MA; Bayoumi A; Al-Khars A; Thulesius O. Adverse drug reaction monitoring in Kuwait (1981-1984). *J Clin Pharmacol.* 25(3): p176-81, Apr 1985.

Muir JW; Besser GM; Edwards CR; Rees LH; Cattell WR; Ackrill P; Baker LR. Bromocriptine improves reduced libido and potency in men receiving maintenance hemodialysis. *Clin Nephrol.* 20(6): p308-14, Dec 1983.

Nagulesparen M; Ang V; Jenkins JS. Bromocriptine treatment of males with pituitary tumours, hyperprolactinaemia, and hypogonadism. *Clin Endocrinol (Oxf).* 9(1): p73-9, Jul 1978.

Okkens AC; van Haaften B; Nickel R. [Fertility problems in the bitch.] Vakgroep Geneeskunde van Gezelschapsdieren, Utrecht. *Tijdschr Diergeneeskd.* 117(8): p229-34, Apr 15 1992.

Pearson D; Shaw S. *Life Extension: A Practical Scientific Approach.* New York: Warner Books, 1982.

*Physicians' Desk Reference (PDR).* Montvale, New Jersey: Medical Economics Data, a division of Medical Economics Company, Inc., 1994.

Perret M; Schilling A. Role of prolactin in a pheromone-like sexual inhibition in the male lesser mouse lemur. *J Endocrinol.* 114(2): p279-87, Aug 1987.

Pierini A.A.; Nusimovich B. Male diabetic sexual impotence: Effects of dopaminergic agents. *Argentina Arch Androl. (USA).* 6(4): p347-50, 1981.

Rigaud P; Jacquet G; Viennet G; Bittard H. [A rare psychogenic anejaculation. Report of a case of prolactin adenoma.] Une etrange anejaculation psychogene. A propos d'un cas d'adenome a prolactine. *Prog Urol (France).* 2(3): p459-63, June 1992.

Schwartz MF; Bauman JE; Masters WH. Hyperprolactinemia and sexual disorders in men. *Biol Psychiatry.* 17(8): p861-76, Aug 1982.

Sobrinho L.G.; Nunes M.C.; Calhaz-Jorge C.; et al. Effect of treatment with bromocriptine on the size and activity of prolactin producing pituitary tumours. *Acta Endocrinol.* 96(1): p24-9, 1981.

Sodersten P; Hansen S; Eneroth P. Inhibition of sexual behaviour in lactating rats. *J Endocrinol.* 99(2): p189-97, Nov 1983.

Sodersten P; Eneroth P J. Effects of exposure to pups on maternal behaviour, sexual behaviour and serum prolactin concentrations in male rats. *Endocrinol.* 102(1): p115-9, Jul 1984.

Staub J.J.; Althaus B.; Wiggli U.; Gratzl O. Drug treatment of hyperprolactinemia and acromegaly. *Schweiz Med Wochenschr (Switzerland).* 113(20): p733-8, 1983.

Stegmayr B; Skogstrom K. Hyperprolactinaemia and testosterone production. Observations in 2 men on long-term dialysis. *Horm Res.* 21(4): p224-8, 1985.

Sullivan G; Lukoff D. Sexual side effects of antipsychotic medication: evaluation and interventions. *Hosp Community Psychiatry.* 41(11): p1238-41, Nov 1990.

Toyokura Y.; Mizuno Y.; Kase M.; et al. Effects of bromocriptine on Parkinsonism. A nation-wide collaborative double-blind study. *J Pn Acta Neurol Scand (DE)*. 72(2): p157-70, 1985.

Tsakok FH; Yong YM; Ng CS. The use of bromocriptine in hyperprolactinemia and galactorrhea in Singapore. *Int J Gynaecol Obstet*. 23(2): p109-13, Apr 1985.

Uitti RJ; Tanner CM; Rajput AH; Goetz CG; Klawans HL; Thiessen. Hypersexuality with antiparkinsonian therapy. *Clin Neuropharmacol*. 12(5): p375-83, Oct 1989.

Van Loon GR. New drugs in the treatment of pituitary disorders. *Prim Care*. 4(4): p721-37, Dec 1977.

Vircburger MI; Prelevic GM; Peric LA; Knezevic J; Djukanovic L J. Testosterone levels after bromocriptine treatment in patients undergoing long-term hemodialysis. *Androl*. 6(2): p113-6, Mar-Apr 1985.

Waddell TG; Ibach DM. Modern chemical aphrodisiacs. *USA Indian J Pharm Sci (India)*. 51(3): p79-82, 1989.

Wass J.A.H.; Thorner M.O.; Morris D.V.; et al. Long term treatment of acromegaly with bromocriptine. *Brit Med J (England)*. 1(6065): p875-8, 1977.

Weizman R; Weizman A; Levi J; Gura V; Zevin D; Maoz B; Wijsenbeek H; Ben David M. Sexual dysfunction associated with hyperprolactinemia in males and females undergoing hemodialysis. *Psychosom Med*. 45(3): p259-69, Jun 1983.

Werder Kv; Fahlbusch R; Landgraf R; Pickardt CR; Rjosk HK; Scriba PC. Treatment of patients with prolactinomas. *J Endocrinol Invest*. 1(1): p47-58, Jan 1978.

Werner S; Hall K; Sjoberg HE. Bromocriptine therapy in patients with acromegaly: effects on growth hormone, somatomedin A and prolactin. *Acta Endocrinol Suppl (Copenh)*. 216: p199-206, 1978.

Winters SJ; Troen P. Altered pulsatile secretion of luteinizing hormone in hypogonadal men with hyperprolactinaemia. *Clin Endocrinol (Oxf)*. 21(3): p257-63, Sep 1984.

## Deprenyl

Block, W. Affects of Bromocriptine on the Brain. *Life Extension Report*. 13(10): p75-8, October 1993.

Dean W; Morgenthaler J; Fowkes S. *Smart Drugs II: The Next Generation*. Petaluma, California: Smart Publications, 1993.

Dilman V; Dean, W. *The Neuroendochrine Theory of Aging & Degenerative Disease*. Pensacola, FL: The Center for Bio-Gerontology, 1992.

Dallo J; Lekka N; Knoll J. The ejaculatory behavior of sexually sluggish male rats treated with (-)deprenyl, apomorphine, bromocriptine and amphetamine *Pol J Pharmacol Pharm Poland*. 38(3): p251-5, 1986.

Dallo J; Yen TT; Knoll J. The aphrodisiac effect of (-)deprenyl in male rats. *Acta Physiol Hung (Hungary)*. 75 Suppl: p75-6, 1990.

Dallo J.; Knoll J. Effect of (-)-para-fluoro-deprenyl on survival and copulation in male rats. *Acta Physiol Hung (Hungary)*.79(2): p125-9, 1992.

Fowkes, S. Deprenyl: The Anti-Aging Drug. *Smart Drug News*. 2(5): Oct 1993. (CERI, POB 4029, Menlo Park, CA, 94026-4029, tel:415-321-2374, fax:415-323-3864)

Fowkes, S. Q&A. *Smart Drug News*. 2(10): Feb 1994. (CERI, POB 4029, Menlo Park, CA, 94026-4029, tel:415-321-2374, fax:415-323-3864)

Knoll J. Deprenyl (selegiline): the history of its development and pharmacological action. *Acta Neurol Scand Suppl (Denmark)*. 95: p57-80, 1983(A).

Knoll J. (-)Deprenyl-medication: A strategy to modulate the age-related decline of the striatal dopaminergic system. *J Am Geriatr Soc (USA)*. 40(8): p839-847, 1992.

Knoll J. [Medical strategy for improving the quality of life in senescence]. Medikamentose Strategie zur Verbesserung der Lebensqualitat in der Seneszenz. *Wien Med Wochenschr Suppl (Austria)*. 98: p1-18, 1986.

Knoll J. The facilitation of dopaminergic activity in the aged brain by (-)deprenyl. A proposal for a strategy to improve the quality of life in senescence. *Mech Ageing Dev (Switzerland)*. 30(2): p109-22, May 13 1985.

Knoll J; Yen TT; Dallo J. Long-lasting, true aphrodisiac effect of (-)-deprenyl in sexually sluggish old male rats. *Mod Probl Pharmacopsychiatry (Switzerland)*. 19: p135-53, 1983(B).

Knoll J; Dallo J; Yen TT. Striatal dopamine, sexual activity and lifespan. Longevity of rats treated with (-)deprenyl. *Life Sci (USA)*. 45(6): p525-31, 1989.

Pearson D; Shaw S. *Durk Pearson & Sandy Shaw's Life Extension Newsletter*. No 2, October 1988.

*Physicians' Desk Reference (PDR)*. Montvale, New Jersey: Medical Economics Data, a division of Medical Economics Company, Inc., 1994.

Rosen RC; Ashton AK. Prosexual Drugs: Empirical status of the 'new aphrodisiacs.' *Archives of Sexual Behavior*. 22(6): p521-43, 1993.

Schatzberg AF; Cole JO. *Manual of Clinical Psychopharmacology, 2nd Edition*. Washington, DC, London, England: American Psychiatric Press Inc. 1990.

Stoessl AJ. Prevention and management of late stage complications in Parkinson's disease. *Can J Neurol Sci (Canada)*.19(1 SUPPL): p113-6, 1992.

Tran Ty Yen; Dallo J; Knoll J. Aphrodisiac action of selective monoamine oxidase inhibitors in male rats. *Kiserl Orvostud (Hungary)*. 33(5): p483-87, 1981.

Yates A; Wolman W. *Aphrodisiacs: Myth and Reality: Medical Aspects of Human Sexuality*. p58-65, Dec 1991.

Yen TT; Dallo J; Knoll J. The aphrodisiac effect of low doses of (-) deprenyl in male rats. *Pol J Pharmacol Pharm (Poland)*. 34(5-6): p303-8, Nov-Dec 1982.

## Other Prosexual Substances

Todd T. Growing Young. *Men's Journal*, October 1994.

Wright K. The Sniff of Legend. *Discover* magazine. 15(4), April 1994.

# Index